Performance Checklists
TO ACCOMPANY

THIRD EDITION

Fundamentals of Nursing

CONCEPTS, PROCESS, AND PRACTICE

ELIZABETH M. MANTYCH, RN, MSN

School of Nursing
University of Missouri—St. Louis
St. Louis, Missouri

PATRICIA A. POTTER, RN, MSN

Director of Nursing Practice
Barnes Hospital
St. Louis, Missouri

ANNE G. PERRY, RN, MSN, EdD

Associate Professor
St. Louis University School of Nursing
St. Louis, Missouri

Printed in the United States of America

Copyright © 1993 by

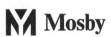 Mosby

St. Louis Baltimore Boston Chicago London Philadelphia Sydney Toronto

Procedures Content

Student _____ Date _____

Instructor _____ Date _____

PERFORMANCE CHECKLIST 5-1 **ADMITTING A CLIENT TO A NURSING DIVISION**

Steps	S	U	Comments
Room Preparation			
1. Wash hands.			
2. Prepare assigned room with needed equipment and supplies.			
3. Prepare bed and adjust to proper position.			
4. Arrange room for client's easy access to bed.			
5. Assemble needed equipment and supplies.			
Admission Process			
6. Greet client and family and introduce yourself.			
7. Escort client and family to assigned room. Introduce roommate if applicable.			
8. Assess client's physical status.			
9. Assess client's and family's psychological status.			
10. Check physician's orders.			
11. Orient client to nursing division.			
12. Assess client's vital signs.			
13. Provide privacy and assist client with undressing and positioning as needed.			
14. Obtain nursing history.			
15. Conduct physical assessment of appropriate body systems.			
16. Instruct client on need for urine specimen, and inform client if other specimens must be obtained.			
17. Inform client about any procedures or treatments scheduled.			
18. Provide opportunity for client's questions.			
19. Collect valuables and complete valuables list.			
20. Allow client and family time together, if desired.			
21. Place call light within reach.			
22. Wash hands.			
23. Record assessment findings on appropriate forms.			
24. Notify physician of client's arrival, reporting any unusual findings.			
25. Begin development of nursing care plan. Confer again with client as needed.			

Student _____ Date _____

Instructor _____ Date _____

PERFORMANCE CHECKLIST 5-2 **DISCHARGING A CLIENT**

Steps	S	U	Comments
Discharge Planning			
1. From time of admission, assess client's health care needs for discharge.	_____	_____	
2. Assess client's and family's need for health teaching related to home setting.	_____	_____	
3. Assess with client and family environmental factors within home setting that may interfere with self-care.	_____	_____	
4. Collaborate with physician and health team members in other disciplines in assessing client's need for referral to receive home health care services.	_____	_____	
5. Assess client's acceptance of health problems and related restrictions.	_____	_____	
6. Consult other health team members about client's needs after discharge. Make appropriate referrals.	_____	_____	
7. Develop and implement nursing plan of care. Evaluate client's progress.	_____	_____	
Preparation Before Day of Discharge			
8. Offer suggestions to change physical arrangement of home to meet client's needs.	_____	_____	
9. Provide client and family with information about community health care resources.	_____	_____	
10. Conduct pertinent teaching sessions with client and family during hospitalization.	_____	_____	
Day of Discharge			
11. Allow client and family to ask questions or discuss issues related to home health care (optional).	_____	_____	
12. Check physician's discharge orders.	_____	_____	
13. Determine whether transportation home has been arranged.	_____	_____	
14. Offer assistance if needed while client dresses and packs belongings.	_____	_____	
15. Check room for belongings. Obtain valuables list and arrange for return of valuables.	_____	_____	
16. Provide client with prescriptions or medications ordered by physician.	_____	_____	
17. Determine if client or family needs to visit agency's business office. If so, make arrangements for them to visit office.	_____	_____	
18. Obtain utility cart for client's belongings and wheelchair, if needed.	_____	_____	
19. Assist client to wheelchair (or stretcher) using proper body mechanics. Escort client to entrance.	_____	_____	
20. Lock wheelchair wheels. Assist client in transferring to vehicle. Assist family with client's personal belongings.	_____	_____	
21. Return to division and notify appropriate department of time of discharge.	_____	_____	

Student _____ Date _____

Instructor _____ Date _____

PERFORMANCE CHECKLIST 18-1 **HANDWASHING**

Steps	S	U	Comments
1. Use easy-to-reach sink with warm running water, soap or disinfectant, and paper towels.	_____	_____	
2. Push wristwatch and uniform sleeves above wrists and remove jewelry.	_____	_____	
3. Keep fingernails short and filed.	_____	_____	
4. Inspect hands for breaks or cuts in skin or cuticles; report lesions when caring for susceptible clients.	_____	_____	
5. Do not let hands or uniform touch sink during washing.	_____	_____	
6. Turn on water using foot and knee pedals; cover handles of hand faucets with paper towel and turn on.	_____	_____	
7. Regulate flow and temperature of water.	_____	_____	
8. Keeping hands and forearms lower than elbows, wet hands and forearms thoroughly with warm running water.	_____	_____	
9. Apply soap to hands; if using bar soap, hold the bar throughout the washing.	_____	_____	
10. Using much lather and friction, wash hands and wrists for 15 to 30 seconds, interlacing fingers and rubbing palms and backs of hands with circular motion.	_____	_____	
11. Clean under fingernails as needed with more soap or clean orangewood stick.	_____	_____	
12. Rinse hands and wrists thoroughly, keeping hands down and elbows up.	_____	_____	
13. Optional: repeat steps 9 through 11, extending the period of washing for 1-, 2-, and 3-minute handwashings.	_____	_____	
14. Dry hands thoroughly, wiping from fingers up to wrists and forearms.	_____	_____	
15. Discard paper towel in proper receptacle.	_____	_____	
16. Turn off faucet with foot and knee pedals; cover hand faucet handles with clean paper towel before touching.	_____	_____	
17. Keep hands and cuticles lubricated with hand lotion or moisturizer.	_____	_____	

Student _____ Date _____

Instructor _____ Date _____

PERFORMANCE CHECKLIST 18-2 **CARING FOR A CLIENT UNDER CATEGORY-SPECIFIC
ISOLATION PRECAUTIONS**

Steps	S	U	Comments
1. Review precautions for isolation category.	————	————	
2. Explain purpose and necessary precautions to client, family, and visitors.	————	————	
3. Assemble necessary equipment and supplies.	————	————	
4. Wash hands.	————	————	
5. Apply gown, mask, and gloves as appropriate.			
a. Apply isolation gown correctly and secure ties at neck and waist.	————	————	
b. Apply disposable gloves with edges overlying gown cuffs.	————	————	
c. Apply surgical mask securely over nose and mouth.	————	————	
6. Enter client's room. Arrange equipment and supplies.	————	————	
7. Assess vital signs.			
a. Place clean paper towel or piece of paper on bedside table.	————	————	
b. Place wristwatch on towel within easy view.	————	————	
c. Assess vital signs, avoiding contact of stethoscope with infective material.	————	————	
d. Record vital signs on clean paper towel or paper.	————	————	
e. Return stethoscope to clean surface after cleaning diaphragm/bell with alcohol.	————	————	
8. Administer medications.			
a. Give oral medication in wrapper or cup.	————	————	
b. Dispose of wrapper or cup in plastic-lined receptacle.	————	————	
c. Administer injection with gloved hand.	————	————	
d. Discard syringe and uncapped needle in special container.	————	————	
e. Place reusable syringe on clean towel for removal and disinfection.	————	————	
9. Administer hygiene.			
a. Prevent gown from becoming wet or soiled.	————	————	
b. Assist client in removing gown; discard in special container.	————	————	
c. Remove bed linen; discard in special container.	————	————	
d. Provide clean bed linen and towels.	————	————	
e. Change gloves, if necessary.	————	————	
10. Collect specimens.			
a. Transfer collected specimen to appropriate container without contaminating container's outer surface.	————	————	
b. Seal containers tightly.	————	————	
c. Label specimens with client's name.	————	————	
d. Transfer specimens correctly into paper bag held by second nurse standing outside room.	————	————	
e. Instruct second nurse on labeling of isolation specimen.	————	————	
f. Send appropriate labeled specimen to laboratory.	————	————	

11. Dispose of linen and trash bags in appropriate containers. _____ _____
12. Resupply room as needed with assistance of care giver at doorway. _____ _____
13. Leave isolation room.
    a. Untie gown at waist; properly remove gloves.
    b. Untie mask strings; drop mask into trash receptacle. _____ _____
    c. Untie neck strings of gown, allowing gown to fall from shoulders. _____ _____
    d. Remove hands from glown sleeve without touching outside of gown. _____ _____
    e. Hold gown inside at shoulder seams and fold inside out; discard in laundry bag. _____ _____
    f. Explain to client when you plan to return. Determine client's needs. _____ _____
    g. Leave room and close door. _____ _____

Student _____ Date _____

Instructor _____ Date _____

PERFORMANCE CHECKLIST 18-3 APPLYING A SURGICAL MASK

Steps	S	U	Comments
1. Locate top edge of mask (usually has thin metal strip).	_____	_____	
2. Hold mask by top two strings or loops.	_____	_____	
3. Tie top two ties at back of head with ties above ears, or slip loops over ears.	_____	_____	
4. Tie two lower ties snugly around neck with mask well under chin.	_____	_____	
5. Gently pinch upper metal band around bridge of nose.	_____	_____	

Student _____

Instructor _____

PERFORMANCE CHECKLIST 18-4 **PREPARING A STERILE FIELD**

Steps	S	U	Comments
1. Select clean work surface above waist level.	——————	——————	
2. Assemble equipment and check dates.	——————	——————	
3. Wash hands.	——————	——————	
4. Open pack.	——————	——————	
5. Pick up folded top of drape with one hand; let it unfold.	——————	——————	
6. Hold drape up and away from the body with both hands.	——————	——————	
7. Position bottom half of drape over work surface.	——————	——————	
8. Allow top half to be placed over work surface last.	——————	——————	
9. Adding sterile items:			
a. Open sterile item.	——————	——————	
b. Peel wrapper; do not allow it to touch sterile field.	——————	——————	
c. Place item onto field at angle.	——————	——————	
d. Dispose of wrapper.	——————	——————	
10. Transferring items with forceps:			
a. Open package with forceps.	——————	——————	
b. Open sterile item.	——————	——————	
c. Grasp handle of forceps; using ends of forceps, grasp sterile item.	——————	——————	
d. Raise sterile item up and over onto sterile field.	——————	——————	
e. Keep handles of forceps outside sterile area.	——————	——————	

Student _____ Date _____

Instructor _____ Date _____

PERFORMANCE CHECKLIST 18-5 SURGICAL HANDWASHING: PREPARING FOR SCRUB

Steps	S	U	Comments
1. Remove all jewelry. Ensure that nails are short and free of polish.			
2. Use deep sink with foot or knee pedals.			
3. Use appropriate antiseptic detergent.			
4. Have two disposable hand brushes and orangestick or disposable nail file available.			
5. Apply cap, covering hair completely.			
6. Apply face mask properly.			
Handwashing			
7. Adjust water flow to lukewarm running flow.			
8. Keeping hands above elbow level throughout the procedure, wet hands and forearms liberally.			
9. Use liberal amount of soap and lather hands and forearms to 5 cm above elbows.			
10. Clean nails with orangestick or file under running water. Discard file.			
11. Wet brush and apply antimicrobial soap. Scrub fingernails, hand, and arm.			
a. Scrub nails (15 strokes).			
b. Using circular motion, scrub palm and anterior surface of fingers (10 strokes).			
c. Scrub side of thumb (10 strokes) and posterior aspect of thumb (10 strokes).			
d. Scrub sides and back of each finger (10 strokes each area).			
e. Scrub back of hand (10 strokes).			
12. Rinse brush thoroughly. Reapply soap.			
13. Mentally divide arms into thirds. Scrub each surface of lower forearm with circular motion (10 strokes); repeat for middle and upper forearm. Discard brush.			
14. With arms flexed, rinse thoroughly from fingertips to elbow in single motion.			
15. Repeat steps 11 to 14 for second arm.			
16. Keeping arms flexed, discard brush. Turn off water with foot pedal. Proceed to operating room.			
17. Pick up sterile towel from top of sterile gown pack. Be sure no one is within arm's reach.			
18. Open towel full length, holding one side away from scrub attire.			
19. Dry each hand and arm separately.			
20. Carefully reverse towel and dry other hand and arm.			
21. Discard towel.			
22. Proceed with sterile gowning.			

Student _____ Date _____

Instructor _____ Date _____

PERFORMANCE CHECKLIST 18-6 **PERFORMING OPEN GLOVING**

Steps	S	U	Comments
1. Have package of proper-sized gloves at treatment area.	——	——	
2. Perform thorough handwashing.	——	——	
3. Peel apart sides of outer package wrapper.	——	——	
4. Lay inner package on clean, flat surface just above waist level.	——	——	
5. Open package, keeping gloves on inside surface of wrapper.	——	——	
6. If gloves are not prepowdered, apply powder lightly to hands over sink or wastebasket.	——	——	
7. Identify right and left gloves; start with dominant hand.	——	——	
8. With thumb and first two fingers of nondominant hand, grasp edge of cut of glove for dominant hand, touching only inside surface.	——	——	
9. Carefully pull glove over dominant hand, ensuring cuff does not roll up wrist.	——	——	
10. With gloved dominant hand, slip fingers underneath second glove's cuff to pick it up.	——	——	
11. Carefully pull second glove over nondominant hand, not allowing gloved hand to touch any part of exposed nondominant hand.	——	——	
12. When both gloves are on, interlock fingers of both hands to secure gloves in position, being careful to touch only sterile sides.	——	——	
Glove disposal			
13. Without touching wrist, grasp outside of one cuff with other gloved hand.	——	——	
14. Pull glove off, turning it inside out. Discard in receptacle.	——	——	
15. Tuck fingers of bare hand inside remaining glove cuff. Discard in receptacle.	——	——	

Student _____ Date _____

Instructor _____ Date _____

PERFORMANCE CHECKLIST 18-7 APPLYING A STERILE GOWN AND PERFORMING CLOSED GLOVING

Steps	S	U	Comments
1. Apply cap, face mask, and foot covers.	————	————	
2. Perform surgical handwashing and dry hands.	————	————	
3. Have circulating nurse open pack containing sterile gown.	————	————	
4. Have circulating nurse prepare glove package.	————	————	
5. Pick up gown at neckline.	————	————	
6. Hold gown at arm's length; allow it to unfold by itself.	————	————	
7. Insert each hand through armholes.	————	————	
8. Have circulating nurse bring gown over shoulders, leaving sleeves covering hands.	————	————	
9. Have circulating nurse tie back of gown at neck and waist.	————	————	
Closed gloving			
10. With hands covered by sleeves, open glove package.	————	————	
11. Pick up glove for dominant hand, with hands covered by sleeve.	————	————	
12. Place glove palm side down on palm of covered hand, with glove fingers pointing toward elbow.	————	————	
13. Using covered nondominant hand, pull glove cuff over dominant hand.	————	————	
14. Grasping top of glove with nondominant hand, extend dominant fingers.	————	————	
15. Repeat steps 11 to 14 to glove nondominant hand.	————	————	
16. Adjust fingers until fully extended into both gloves.	————	————	
17. For wraparound sterile gowns, release front fastener.	————	————	
18. Handing tie to stationary team member, turn 360 degrees to left and secure tie to gown.	————	————	

PERFORMANCE CHECKLIST 19-1   **MEASURING BODY TEMPERATURE**

Steps	S	U	Comments
1. Assess client for signs and symptoms of alterations in body temperature.	————	————	
2. Explain procedure and purpose to client.	————	————	
3. For oral temperature, wait 30 minutes before taking if client has smoked or ingested foods or liquids.	————	————	
4. Prepare needed equipment and supplies.	————	————	
5. Wash hands.	————	————	
6. **Oral temperature—electronic thermometer**			
a. Assist client to comfortable, convenient position.	————	————	
b. Attach oral probe (blue tip) to thermometer and grasp top of stem.	————	————	
c. Slide plastic probe cover over probe until it locks.	————	————	
d. Place probe under tongue in posterior sublingual pocket.	————	————	
e. Have client hold thermometer with lips closed.	————	————	
f. Leave probe in place until audible signal occurs. Temperature appears on digital display.	————	————	
g. Remove probe; inform client of reading.	————	————	
h. Push ejection buttton and discard plastic probe cover.	————	————	
i. Return probe to storage well.	————	————	
j. Remove and dispose of gloves. Wash hands.	————	————	
k. Return thermometer to charger unit.	————	————	
7. **Oral temperature—glass thermometer**			
a. Assist client to comfortable, convenient position.	————	————	
b. Properly hold thermometer and rinse in cold water if needed.	————	————	
c. Wipe thermometer with tissue from bulb end toward fingers; dispose of tissue.	————	————	
d. Read mercury level and shake down if necessary.	————	————	
e. Gently place thermometer in posterior sublingual pocket.	————	————	
f. Ask client to hold thermometer with lips closed.	————	————	
g. Leave thermometer in place 2 to 8 minutes or according to agency policy.	————	————	
h. Carefully remove thermometer and read at eye level; inform client of reading.	————	————	
i. Wipe thermometer with soft tissue and dispose of tissue.	————	————	
j. Wash, rinse, and dry thermometer, store properly.	————	————	
k. Remove and dispose of gloves. Wash hands.	————	————	
8. **Rectal temperature—electronic thermometer**			
a. Provide privacy. Cover client's upper body and lower extremities with sheet.	————	————	
b. Assist client to Sim's position. Expose anal area.	————	————	
c. Attach rectal probe (red tip) to thermometer unit.	————	————	
d. Grasp top of stem and slide plastic probe cover over thermometer probe until it locks.	————	————	
e. Apply disposable gloves.	————	————	

f. Ask client to breathe slowly and relax.   _____   _____

g. Expose anus with nondominant hand and insert thermometer 1.2 cm for infant and 3.5 cm for adult.   _____   _____

h. Withdraw thermometer immediately if resistance is felt.   _____   _____

i. Hold probe in place until audible signal occurs.   _____   _____

j. Read temperature on digital display.   _____   _____

k. Remove probe and inform client of reading.   _____   _____

l. Push ejection button and discard plastic probe cover.   _____   _____

m. Return probe to storage well.   _____   _____

n. Wipe anal area to remove feces. Remove and dispose of gloves.   _____   _____

o. Return client to comfortable position.   _____   _____

p. Wash hands.   _____   _____

9. Rectal temperature—glass thermometer

a. Provide privacy. Cover client's upper body and lower extremities with sheet.   _____   _____

b. Have adult assume Sims' position; child, the prone position. Expose anal area.   _____   _____

c. Prepare thermometer following steps 7b to 7d.   _____   _____

d. Apply lubricant to thermometer with tissue.   _____   _____

e. Apply disposable gloves.   _____   _____

f. Expose anus with nondominant hand and insert thermometer 1.2 cm for infant and 3.5 cm for adult.   _____   _____

g. Remove thermometer if resistance is felt.   _____   _____

h. Leave thermometer in place 2 minutes or according to agency policy.   _____   _____

i. Carefully remove thermometer.   _____   _____

j. Wipe thermometer with tissue and dispose of tissue.   _____   _____

k. Read thermometer at eye level; inform client of reading.   _____   _____

l. Wipe anal area to remove lubricant and feces.   _____   _____

m. Help client tto comfortable position.   _____   _____

n. Wash, rinse, and dry thermometer; store properly.   _____   _____

o. Dispose of gloves. Wash hands.   _____   _____

10. Axillary temperature—electronic thermometer

a. Provide privacy.   _____   _____

b. Position client lying supine or sitting.   _____   _____

c. Move clothing away from shoulder and arm.   _____   _____

d. Prepare electronic thermometer by following steps 6b and 6c.   _____   _____

e. Insert probe into center of axilla, lower client's arm, and place arm over chest.   _____   _____

f. Hold probe in place until audible signal occurs.   _____   _____

g. Read temperature on digital display.   _____   _____

h. Remove probe from axilla; inform client of reading.   _____   _____

i. Push ejection button and discard plastic probe cover.   _____   _____

j. Return electronic probe to storage well.   _____   _____

k. Replace client's clothing or gown.   _____   _____

l. Position client comfortably.   _____   _____

m. Wash hands.   _____   _____

11. Axillary temperature—glass thermometer

a. Provide privacy.   _____   _____

b. Position client lying supine or sitting; move clothing or gown away from shoulder and arm.   _____   _____

c. Prepare thermometer by following steps 7b to 7d.   _____   _____

d. Insert thermometer into center of axilla, lower client's arm over thermometer, and place arm across chest.   _____   _____

e. Hold thermometer in place for 5 to 10 minutes.   _____   _____

f. Remove thermometer and wipe it off with tissue. Dispose of tissue.   _____   _____

g. Read thermometer at eye level; inform client of reading.

h. Properly wash, rinse, and dry thermometer; store properly.

i. Help client to replace clothing or gown.

j. Wash hands.

12. **Tympanic membrane thermometer**

a. Attach tympanic probe cover to thermometer unit.

b. Insert probe into ear canal with gentle pressure.

c. Remove thermometer after reading is displayed on digital unit, approximately 2 seconds.

d. Remove probe cover and place in proper receptacle.

e. Return thermometer to storage unit.

f. Wash hands.

13. Compare temperature reading with client's baseline and normal range for age group.

14. Repeat procedure if temperature is abnormal.

15. Properly record procedure and observations and report abnormal findings.

Temp

Timpanic + ORAL - 98.6 - 2.8 min / 2 sec temp. · Oral

Rectal - 99.6 - 2 min

Axillary - 97.6 - 5-10 min

Factors affect change: Smoking
Exercise
Metabolism
Age
Hormonal Level
Stress - ~~with force~~ -
Environment
Smoking - 30 sec

Chills - trying to conserve heat.

Surgical Patients - usually use rectal temp

Pulse
Strength (Quality)
Rhythm
Rate

PERFORMANCE CHECKLIST 19-2 **ASSESSING PULSE RATE**

Steps	S	U	Comments
1. Assess factors that influence pulse character.	————	————	
2. Explain procedure to client and encourage relaxation.	————	————	
3. Prepare equipment and supplies.	————	————	
4. Wash hands.	————	————	
5. **Radial pulse**			
a. Place client's forearm across chest, wrist extended if supine, or with elbow bent 90 degrees, wrist extended with palm down if sitting.	————	————	
b. Place first two fingers along radial artery and gently compress against the radius.	————	————	
c. Obliterate pulse briefly and relax pressure so pulse is palpable.	————	————	
d. Observe second hand of watch and count pulse for 30 seconds and multiply by 2 (if regular) or count for 60 seconds (if irregular).	————	————	
e. Assess rhythm of pulse.	————	————	
f. Asses pulse strength.	————	————	
g. Palpate elasticity of arterial wall.	————	————	
h. Assist client to comfortable position.	————	————	
i. Discuss findings with client.	————	————	
6. **Apical pulse**			
a. Properly clean stethoscope.	————	————	
b. Assist client to supine or sitting position.	————	————	
c. Expose sternum and left side of chest.	————	————	
d. Properly palpate angle of Louis; palpate second intercostal space; proceed downward to the fifth intercostal space; palpate point of maximum impulse (PMI).	————	————	
e. Warm diaphragm of stethoscope in palm of hand for 5 to 10 seconds.	————	————	
f. Place diaphragm over PMI and auscultate for normal S_1 and S_2 heart sounds.	————	————	
g. Using second hand of watch, begin to count rate for 30 seconds and multiply by 2 (if regular) or count for 60 seconds (if irregular).	————	————	
h. Assess rhythm of pulse.	————	————	
i. Position client comfortably.	————	————	
j. Discuss findings with client.	————	————	
7. Wash hands.	————	————	
8. Compare pulse rate with client's previous baseline and normal range for that age group.	————	————	
9. Properly record procedure and observations.	————	————	

Popliteal – behind knee, carotid, brachial, apical femoral, Dorsalis pedis

PERFORMANCE CHECKLIST 19-3 **ASSESSING RESPIRATIONS**

Steps	S	U	Comments
1. Assess factors that may affect respirations.	———	———	
2. Wait 5 to 10 minutes before assessing respiration for client who has been active.	———	———	
3. Position client comfortably.	———	———	
4. Prepare needed equipment and supplies.	———	———	
5. If needed, move bed linen or gown to expose chest.	———	———	
6. Position client's arm across abdomen or lower chest.	———	———	
7. Place own hand over client's upper abdomen.	———	———	
8. Observe complete respiratory cycle (one inspiration and one expiration).	———	———	
9. Observe second hand of watch and count number of respirations in 30 seconds and multiply by 2; with child or in adult with irregular respirations, count for 60 seconds.	———	———	
10. Assess whether depth of respiration is shallow, normal, or deep.	———	———	
11. Assess rhythm of ventilatory cycle.	———	———	
12. Replace gown and bed linen.	———	———	
13. Wash hands.	———	———	
14. Discuss findings with client.	———	———	
15. Compare respirations with client's previous baseline and normal rate for that age group.	———	———	
16. Properly record procedure and observations.	———	———	

Resp- 12-20 resp

Even

Rate, Rhythm + quality
        deep/shallow

deep + regular = normal

PERFORMANCE CHECKLIST 19-4   ASSESSING BLOOD PRESSURE BY AUSCULTATION

Steps	S	U	Comments
1. Assess for factors that may influence blood pressure.			
2. Determine best site for assessment.			
3. Prepare equipment and supplies.			
4. Ask client to avoid activity and smoking for 30 minutes before assessment.			
5. Assist client to sitting or lying position.			
6. Explain procedure to client.			
7. Wash hands.			
8. Support client's forearm at heart level with palm up.			
9. Expose upper arm.			
10. Palpate brachial artery.			
11. Position cuff 2.5 cm above brachial artery pulsation.			
12. Center arrows on cuff over brachial artery.			
13. Wrap fully deflated cuff evenly and snugly around upper arm.			
14. Position manometer at eye level.			
15. Palpate brachial or radial artery while inflating cuff to pressure above point at which radial artery pulsation disappears.			
16. Deflate cuff and wait 30 seconds.			
17. Prepare to listen through the stethoscope.			
18. Place diaphragm or bell over brachial artery.			
19. Tighten pressure valve and inflate cuff to pressure level 30 mm Hg above palpated systolic pressure.			
20. Slowly release valve to allow mercury to fall 2 to 3 mm Hg per second.			
21. Note point on manometer when first clear sound is heard.			
22. Continue to deflate cuff, noting point at which muffled sound occurs and point at which it disappears.			
23. Deflate cuff rapidly and remove from client's arm.			
24. If first client assessment, repeat procedure on other arm and compare with first assessment.			
25. Assist client to comfortable position.			
26. Inform client of reading.			
27. Wash hands.			
28. Compare readings with client's baseline and normal average for that age group.			
29. Record procedure and observations properly.			
30. Report immediately any significant change from normal readings.			

Student _____ Date _____

Instructor _____ Date _____

PERFORMANCE CHECKLIST 21-1   ADMINISTERING ORAL MEDICATIONS

Steps	S	U	Comments
1. Assess client for contraindications.	_____	_____	
2. Determine client's preference for fluids.	_____	_____	
3. Prepare needed supplies and equipment.	_____	_____	
4. Check each medication card listing prescribed medications and times for accuracy by comparing it with physician's written medication order: right client, drug, dosage, route, and time of administration.	_____	_____	
5. Prepare medications.			
a. Wash hands.	_____	_____	
b. Arrange tray and cups. Prepare medications for one client at a time, keeping medication forms for client together and separate from forms for other clients.	_____	_____	
c. Select correct medication and check against medication card.	_____	_____	
d. Calculate and double-check correct dosage of each medication.	_____	_____	
e. Pour correct number of tablets, capsules, or packaged unit-dose tablets or capsules into cup, avoiding contact with fingers.	_____	_____	
f. Grind tablets in mortar with pestle.	_____	_____	
g. Pour liquids correctly: remove bottle cap and place it upside down; hold bottle correctly and pour at eye level into cup; discard excess liquid into sink; and wipe lip of bottle with paper towel before replacing cap.	_____	_____	
h. For narcotic medications, check and sign narcotic record for drug count.	_____	_____	
i. Again, compare prepared drug with medication form.	_____	_____	
j. Replace unused unit doses or stock containers, checking labels a third time. Place medications and forms together on cart.	_____	_____	
6. Administer medications.			
a. Take medications together on tray or cart to client at proper time.	_____	_____	
b. Identify client by comparing name on card or form with client's identification band and by asking client his or her full name.	_____	_____	
c. Perform necessary preadministration assessment.	_____	_____	
d. Explain medication's action and purpose to client.	_____	_____	
e. Assist client to sitting or side-lying position.	_____	_____	
f. Correctly administer medication, offering liquid with drugs to be swallowed.	_____	_____	
g. If client is unable to hold medication, place cup to lips and gently introduce medication into the mouth one pill or capsule at a time.	_____	_____	
h. Discard and replace any tablet or capsule that falls to the floor.	_____	_____	
i. Stay with client until each medication has been swallowed.	_____	_____	
j. Assist client in returning to comfortable position.	_____	_____	
k. Discard used supplies and wash hands.	_____	_____	
7. Correctly record medication and return record to appropriate place.	_____	_____	
8. Return within 30 minutes to evaluate client's response.	_____	_____	

Student _____ Date _____

Instructor _____ Date _____

PERFORMANCE CHECKLIST 21-2 **PREPARING INJECTIONS FROM AMPULES AND VIALS**

Steps	S	U	Comments
1. Wash hands.	_____	_____	
2. Prepare needed equipment and supplies and assemble at work area in medicine room.	_____	_____	
3. **Prepare injection from ampule.**			
a. Tap top of ampule lightly and quickly with finger.	_____	_____	
b. Place gauze pad or dry swab around neck of ampule.	_____	_____	
c. Snap neck of ampule away from hands.	_____	_____	
d. Draw up medication quickly.	_____	_____	
e. Hold ampule upside down or place on flat surface.	_____	_____	
f. Insert needle into center of ampule opening; do not touch rim.	_____	_____	
g. Aspirate medication into syringe, tipping the ampule to keep liquid within reach of needle.	_____	_____	
h. Do not expel aspirated air bubbles back into ampule; remove needle from ampule; eject air.	_____	_____	
i. Expel excess fluid into sink.	_____	_____	
j. Change and cover needle with sheath or cap; dispose of soiled supplies; properly dispose of ampule.	_____	_____	
4. **Prepare injection from vial.**			
a. Remove metal cap of vial to expose rubber seal.	_____	_____	
b. Wipe off surface of rubber seal with alcohol swab.	_____	_____	
c. Remove needle cap of syringe and pull back on the plunger to draw air into syringe equivalent to amount of medication to be aspirated.	_____	_____	
d. Insert needle tip with bevel pointing up through center of rubber seal.	_____	_____	
e. Inject air into vial, grasping plunger.	_____	_____	
f. Invert vial held between thumb and fingers of nondominant hand, grasping barrel and plunger with thumb and forefinger of dominant hand.	_____	_____	
g. Keep tip of needle below fluid level and allow air pressure to fill syringe with medication.	_____	_____	
h. Pull back plunger to obtain correct amount of medication in syringe, if necessary.	_____	_____	
i. Tap syringe barrel to dislodge any air bubbles; expel them into vial.	_____	_____	
j. Remove needle from vial.	_____	_____	
k. Expel remaining air.	_____	_____	
l. Change needle and cover.	_____	_____	
m. For multidose vial, make label with necessary information.	_____	_____	
n. Dispose of soiled supplies.	_____	_____	
5. Clean work area. Wash hands.	_____	_____	
6. Check fluid level in syringe and compare with desired dosage.	_____	_____	

Student _____ Date _____

Instructor _____ Date _____

PERFORMANCE CHECKLIST 21-3 **ADMINISTERING INJECTIONS**

Steps	S	U	Comments
1. Assess indications for proper route for injecting medication.	_____	_____	
2. Assess client's medical history and attitude toward receiving medication.	_____	_____	
3. Wash hands.	_____	_____	
4. Prepare needed equipment and supplies.	_____	_____	
5. Check medication order.	_____	_____	
6. Identify client.	_____	_____	
7. Prepare correct dosage of medication from ampule or vial.	_____	_____	
8. Expel all air. For IM injection, prepare an air lock if needed.	_____	_____	
9. Apply disposable gloves.	_____	_____	
10. Explain procedure to client.	_____	_____	
11. Provide privacy.	_____	_____	
12. Avoid unnecessary exposure.	_____	_____	
13. Select appropriate injection site. Assess for bruises, edema, masses, tenderness, or discolorations.	_____	_____	
14. Rotate sites if indicated.	_____	_____	
15. Assist client to appropriate comfortable position.	_____	_____	
16. Relocate injection site using anatomical landmarks.	_____	_____	
17. Cleanse site properly with antiseptic swab.	_____	_____	
18. Remove needle cap.	_____	_____	
19. Hold syringe between thumb and forefinger of dominant hand in proper position for type of injection chosen.	_____	_____	
20. Administer injection.	_____	_____	
21. **SQ injections**			
a. For average-sized client, spread skin tightly across injection site or pinch skin with nondominant hand.	_____	_____	
b. Inject needle quickly and firmly at 45-degree angle.	_____	_____	
c. For obese client, pinch skin at site and inject needle below skin fold.	_____	_____	
22. **IM injections**			
a. Position nondominant hand at anatomical landmark and spread skin tightly.	_____	_____	
b. Inject needle quickly at 90-degree angle.	_____	_____	
c. For clients with small muscle mass, grasp body of muscle between thumb and other fingers.	_____	_____	
23. **ID injections**			
a. With nondominant hand, stretch skin over site with thumb or forefinger.	_____	_____	
b. With needle almost against client's skin, insert it at 5- to 15-degree angle until resistance is felt; advance needle approximately 3 mm below skin surface.	_____	_____	
24. When needle has entered site of SQ or IM injection only, grasp lower end of syringe barrel with nondominant hand; avoid moving syringe.	_____	_____	
25. With dominant hand, slowly pull back on plunger to aspirate medication.	_____	_____	

26. If blood appears in syringe, withdraw needle and repeat procedure. _____ _____
27. Inject medication slowly. _____ _____
28. Note formation of small bleb on skin's surface during ID injection. _____ _____
29. Withdraw needle while applying alcohol swab above or over injection site. _____ _____
30. For SQ or IM injections only, massage skin lightly. _____ _____
31. Assist client to comfortable position. _____ _____
32. Discard needle and syringe appropriately. _____ _____
33. Wash hands. _____ _____
34. Return to client and ask about sensations at injection site; observe for allergic reaction after ID injection. _____ _____
35. Return to evaluate response to medication in 10 to 30 minutes. _____ _____
36. Draw circle around perimeter of injection site for ID injection. _____ _____
37. For SQ and IM injections, chart dosage, route, site, and time; record properly. _____ _____
38. For ID injections, record area of injection, amount and type of substance, and date and time. _____ _____

Student _____ Date _____

Instructor _____ Date _____

PERFORMANCE CHECKLIST 21-4 ADDING MEDICATIONS TO INTRAVENOUS FLUID CONTAINERS

Steps	S	U	Comments
1. Check physician's order.	————	————	
2. Assess for drug compatibility if more than one medication is to be added.	————	————	
3. Prepare needed equipment and supplies.	————	————	
4. Identify client.	————	————	
5. Explain procedure to client. Encourage client to report discomfort.	————	————	
6. Wash hands.	————	————	
7. Assemble supplies in medication room.	————	————	
8. Prepare medication from vial or ampule.	————	————	
9. Adding medication to new container:			
a. Locate injection port on IV solution bag or site on IV bottle and remove port cover.	————	————	
b. Wipe port or injection site with alcohol or antiseptic swab.	————	————	
c. Insert needle of syringe through center of port or injection site and inject medication.	————	————	
d. Withdraw syringe.	————	————	
e. Mix solution by gently turning container.	————	————	
f. Complete medication label and place upside down on container.	————	————	
g. Spike and hang container. Regulate infusion rate.	————	————	
10. Adding medication to existing container:			
a. Prepare vented IV container.	————	————	
b. Check remaining volume of solution.	————	————	
c. Verify dilution of medication desired.	————	————	
d. Close IV infusion clamp.	————	————	
e. Wipe medication port with alcohol or antiseptic swab.	————	————	
f. Inject medication through injection port.	————	————	
g. Gently mix solution.	————	————	
h. Rehang bag and regulate infusion rate.	————	————	
i. Complete and affix medication label.	————	————	
11. Properly dispose of equipment and supplies.	————	————	
12. Wash hands.	————	————	
13. Correctly record medication; report any side effects.	————	————	

Student _____ Date _____

Instructor _____ Date _____

PERFORMANCE CHECKLIST 21-5 ADMINISTERING INTRAVENOUS MEDICATIONS BY PIGGYBACK OR VOLUME-CONTROL ADMINISTRATION SETS

Steps	S	U	· Comments
1. Check physician's order for type of solution, medication, and dosage.	———	———	
2. Assess patency of IV line.	———	———	
3. Assess site for signs of infiltration or phlebitis.	———	———	
4. Prepare needed equipment and supplies.	———	———	
5. Wash hands.	———	———	
6. Identify client.	———	———	
7. **Administer medications by piggyback set.**			
a. Assemble supplies in medication room.	———	———	
b. Connect infusion tubing to medication bag.	———	———	
c. Hang medication bag at or above level of main bag.	———	———	
d. Connect needle to end of infusion tubing.	———	———	
e. Identify client.	———	———	
f. Cleanse injection port of main line with antiseptic swab.	———	———	
g. Insert needle of secondary line through injection port of main line; regulate appropriate flow rate of medication solution.	———	———	
h. After infusion of medication, turn off flow regulator on secondary line.	———	———	
i. Regulate main line if necessary.	———	———	
j. Leave secondary needle, tubing, and bag in place for future use or discard appropriately.	———	———	
8. **Administer medications by volume-control set (e.g., Volutrol).**			
a. Assemble supplies in medication room.	———	———	
b. Prepare medication from vial or ampule.	———	———	
c. Identify client.	———	———	
d. Fill Volutrol with desired amount of fluid by opening clamp between Volutrol and main IV bag.	———	———	
e. Cleanse injection port on top with antiseptic swab.	———	———	
f. Insert syringe needle into port and inject medication.	———	———	
g. Gently rotate Volutrol between hands to mix medication with solution.	———	———	
h. Regulate appropriate infusion rate.	———	———	
i. Label Volutrol.	———	———	
j. Properly dispose of needle and syringe.	———	———	
9. Observe client for signs of adverse reactions.	———	———	
10. During infusion, periodically check infusion rate and IV site.	———	———	
11. Correctly record medication; record fluid volumes on intake and output form.	———	———	

Student _____ Date _____

Instructor _____ Date _____

PERFORMANCE CHECKLIST 21-6 **ADMINISTERING MEDICATIONS BY INTRAVENOUS BOLUS (PUSH)**

Steps	S	U	Comments
1. Check physician's medication order.	————	————	
2. Wash hands.	————	————	
3. Assemble and prepare equipment and supplies.	————	————	
4. Identify client.	————	————	
5. Determine that IV fluids are infusing at proper rate.	————	————	
6. **Existing line**			
a. Select injection port of tubing closest to needle insertion site.	————	————	
b. Cleanse injection port with antiseptic swab.	————	————	
c. Withdraw syringe.	————	————	
d. Mix solution by gently turning container.	————	————	
e. Rehang container and check infusion rate.	————	————	
7. **Intravenous lock**			
a. Assemble all equipment and supplies.	————	————	
b. Cleanse heparin lock's rubber diaphragm with antiseptic swab.	————	————	
c. Insert 25-gauge needle of syringe containing medication through center of diaphragm.	————	————	
d. Using watch with second hand, inject medication bolus slowly over several minutes, according to package directions.	————	————	
e. Withdraw syringe.	————	————	
f. Insert needle of syringe containing diluted heparin (flush) solution and inject solution.	————	————	
g. Observe client closely for adverse reactions.	————	————	
8. Dispose of needles and syringes.	————	————	
9. Wash hands.	————	————	
10. Record drug, dosage, route, and time administered on form.			

Student _____ Date _____

Instructor _____ Date _____

PERFORMANCE CHECKLIST 21-7 **ADMINISTERING EYEDROPS AND OINTMENT**

Steps	S	U	Comments
1. Review medication order.	————	————	
2. Identify client.	————	————	
3. Assess external eye structures.	————	————	
4. Wash hands.	————	————	
5. Prepare equipment and supplies.	————	————	
6. Explain procedure to client.	————	————	
7. Arrange supplies at bedside.	————	————	
8. Position client supine or in chair with head slightly hyperextended.	————	————	
9. Remove any crusts or drainage from eyelid margins or inner canthus.	————	————	
10. Hold cotton ball or tissue in nondominant hand just below lower eyelid.	————	————	
11. Gently pressing against bony orbit (not eyeball), press downward.	————	————	
12. Ask client to look upward.	————	————	
13. Instill eyedrops.			
a. Hold eyedropper in dominant hand 1 to 2 cm above conjunctival sac and drop prescribed number of medication drops into conjunctival sac.	————	————	
b. Any drops landing on outer margins or blinked out of eye must be repeated.	————	————	
c. For drugs having systemic effects, cover finger with clean tissue and apply gentle pressure to nasolacrimal duct for 30 to 60 seconds.	————	————	
d. Ask client to close eye.	————	————	
14. Instill eye ointment.			
a. With ointments, apply thin stream evenly along inside edge of lower eyelid, on conjunctiva.	————	————	
b. Ask client to look down.	————	————	
c. Apply thin stream along upper lid margin on conjunctiva.	————	————	
d. Have client close eye and rub lid lightly with cotton ball in circular motion.	————	————	
15. Wipe any excess medication gently from inner to outer canthus.	————	————	
16. Apply clean eye patch, if used.	————	————	
17. Dispose of soiled supplies; wash hands.	————	————	
18. Observe client for signs of adverse reaction.	————	————	
19. Correctly record medication.	————	————	

Student _____ Date _____

Instructor _____ Date _____

PERFORMANCE CHECKLIST 21-8 ADMINISTERING EARDROPS

Steps	S	U	Comments
1. Review physician's order.	____	____	
2. Identify client.	____	____	
3. Assess external ear structures and canal.	____	____	
4. Wash hands.	____	____	
5. Prepare equipment and supplies.	____	____	
6. Explain procedure to client.	____	____	
7. Arrange supplies at bedside.	____	____	
8. Position client in side-lying position with ear to be treated facing up.	____	____	
9. If cerumen occludes outermost part of ear canal, wipe out gently with cotton-tipped applicator.	____	____	
10. Straighten ear canal by pulling pinna down and back (children) or upward and outward (adults).	____	____	
11. Holding dropper 1 cm above ear canal, instill prescribed drops.	____	____	
12. With client remaining in side-lying position 2 to 3 minutes, apply gentle pressure to tragus with finger.	____	____	
13. If ordered, position cotton ball in outermost part of ear canal for 15 minutes.	____	____	
14. Dispose of soiled supplies. Wash hands.	____	____	
15. Assist client to comfortable position.	____	____	
16. Evaluate condition of external ear.	____	____	
17. Correctly record medication administered on medication form; record condition of ear canal in nurses' notes.	____	____	

Student _____ Date _____

Instructor _____ Date _____

PERFORMANCE CHECKLIST 21-9 ADMINISTERING NASAL DROPS

Steps	S	U	Comments
1. Review physician's order.	_____	_____	
2. Determine from record which sinus is affected.	_____	_____	
3. Identify client.	_____	_____	
4. Assess condition of nose and sinuses.	_____	_____	
5. Wash hands.	_____	_____	
6. Prepare needed equipment and supplies.	_____	_____	
7. Explain procedure to client.	_____	_____	
8. Arrange supplies at bedside.	_____	_____	
9. Unless contraindicated, ask client to blow nose.	_____	_____	
10. Administer nasal drops.			
a. Assist client to supine position.	_____	_____	
b. For posterior pharynx, tilt head backward.	_____	_____	
c. For ethmoid or sphenoid sinuses, tilt head back over edge of bed or place pillow under shoulders.	_____	_____	
d. For frontal and maxillary sinuses, tilt head back over bed or pillow and tilt toward side to be treated.	_____	_____	
e. Have client breathe through mouth.	_____	_____	
f. Hold dropper 1 cm above nares and instill prescribed number of drops toward midline of ethmoid bone.	_____	_____	
g. Have client maintain supine position for 5 minutes.	_____	_____	
h. Offer tissue for runny nose but caution against blowing for several minutes.	_____	_____	
11. Assist client to comfortable position.	_____	_____	
12. Dispose of soiled supplies and wash hands.	_____	_____	
13. Observe client for side effects 15 to 30 minutes after procedure.	_____	_____	
14. Correctly record medication.	_____	_____	

Student _____ Date _____

Instructor _____ Date _____

PERFORMANCE CHECKLIST 21-10 ADMINISTERING VAGINAL INSTILLATIONS

Steps	S	U	Comments
1. Review physician's order.	___	___	
2. Identify client.	___	___	
3. Inspect external genitalia and vaginal canal.	___	___	
4. Wash hands.	___	___	
5. Prepare needed equipment and supplies.	___	___	
6. Explain procedure to client.	___	___	
7. Arrange supplies at bedside.	___	___	
8. Provide privacy.	___	___	
9. Assist client to dorsal recumbent position.	___	___	
10. Keep abdomen and lower extremities draped.	___	___	
11. Apply disposable gloves.	___	___	
12. Provide adequate lighting.	___	___	
13. **Suppository insertion with gloved hand**			
a. Take suppository from wrapper and lubricate smooth or rounded end.	___	___	
b. Lubricate gloves.	___	___	
c. Retract labial folds with nondominant gloved hand.	___	___	
d. Insert rounded end of suppository 7.5 to 10 cm along posterior wall of vagina.	___	___	
e. Wipe away lubricant from orifice and labia.	___	___	
14. **Suppository insertion by applicator**			
a. Take suppository from wrapper and lubricate rounded end.	___	___	
b. With plunger out, place pointed tip of suppository on end of applicator.	___	___	
c. Retract labial folds with nondominant gloved hand.	___	___	
d. With dominant gloved hand, advance applicator 5 to 7.5 cm along posterior vaginal wall; push plunger to deposit suppository.	___	___	
e. Withdraw and place applicator on paper towel; wipe lubricant from orifice and labia.	___	___	
15. **Application of cream**			
a. Fill cream applicator.	___	___	
b. Retract labial folds with nondominant gloved hand.	___	___	
c. With dominant gloved hand, insert applicator 5 to 7.5 cm; push plunger.	___	___	
d. Withdraw and place applicator on paper towel; wipe lubricant from orifice and labia.	___	___	
16. Remove gloves properly and discard in appropriate container. Wash hands.	___	___	
17. Tell client to remain flat on her back for at least 10 minutes.	___	___	
18. Wash applicator, if used, and store for future use. Wash hands.	___	___	
19. Offer client perineal pad.	___	___	
20. Inspect condition of vaginal canal and external genitalia between applications.	___	___	
21. Correctly record medication.	___	___	

Student _____ Date _____

Instructor _____ Date _____

PERFORMANCE CHECKLIST 21-11 ADMINISTERING RECTAL SUPPOSITORIES

Steps	S	U	Comments
1. Check physician's order.	_____	_____	
2. Identify client.	_____	_____	
3. Review client's medical record.	_____	_____	
4. Examine external condition of anus; palpate rectal walls.	_____	_____	
5. Wash and glove hands.	_____	_____	
6. Prepare needed equipment and supplies.	_____	_____	
7. Explain procedure to client.	_____	_____	
8. Arrange supplies at bedside.	_____	_____	
9. Provide privacy.	_____	_____	
10. Position client in side-lying position with upper leg flexed upward.	_____	_____	
11. Keep client draped except for anal area.	_____	_____	
12. Correctly apply disposable gloves (if previous pair is soiled).	_____	_____	
13. Remove suppository from wrapper and lubricate rounded end with jelly.	_____	_____	
14. Lubricate gloved index finger of dominant hand.	_____	_____	
15. Ask client to take slow, deep breaths through mouth and relax anal sphincter.	_____	_____	
16. Retract client's buttocks with nondominant hand.	_____	_____	
17. With index finger of dominant hand, gently insert suppository through anus, past internal sphincter, and against rectal wall, 10 cm (adults) or 5 cm (children, infants).	_____	_____	
18. Withdraw finger and wipe anal area clean.	_____	_____	
19. Remove and dispose of gloves.	_____	_____	
20. Keep client flat or on side for 5 minutes.	_____	_____	
21. If suppository contains laxative or fecal softener, be sure client can receive help to reach bedpan or toilet.	_____	_____	
22. Wash hands.	_____	_____	
23. Return in 5 minutes to determine if suppository has been expelled.	_____	_____	
24. Correctly record medication.	_____	_____	

Student _____ Date _____

Instructor _____ Date _____

PERFORMANCE CHECKLIST 21-12 **USING METERED-DOSE INHALERS**

Steps	S	U	Comments
1. Assess client's ability to use inhaler.	____	____	
2. Check drug schedule.	____	____	
3. Show client how to prepare equipment and supplies.	____	____	
4. Encourage client to assume comfortable position.	____	____	
5. Allow client to handle inhaler and canister; explain how they fit together.	____	____	
6. Explain metered doses; caution client about overuse and side effects.	____	____	
7. Demonstrate steps used to administer dose.	____	____	
a. Remove cap and hold inhaler upright.	____	____	
b. Shake inhaler.	____	____	
c. Tilt head back slightly and breathe out.	____	____	
d. Position inhaler by one of the following ways:			
(1) Open mouth with inhaler 1 to 2 inches away.	____	____	
(2) Attach spacer to mouthpiece of inhaler and place mouth on spacer.	____	____	
(3) Place inhaler in mouth.	____	____	
e. Press down on inhaler to release medication while inhaling slowly.	____	____	
f. Breathe slowly for 2 to 3 seconds.	____	____	
g. Hold breath for approximately 10 seconds.	____	____	
h. Repeat puffs as ordered, waiting 1 minute between puffs.	____	____	
8. Instruct client to follow physician's orders on intervals between inhalations.	____	____	
9. Explain sensations to be expected.	____	____	
10. Show client how to remove and clean inhaler.	____	____	
11. Have client demonstrate use of inhaler and explain drug schedule.	____	____	
12. Instruct client against repeating inhalations before scheduled dose.	____	____	
13. Describe skills taught and client's ability to perform procedure in nurses' notes.	____	____	

Student _____ Date _____

Instructor _____ Date _____

PERFORMANCE CHECKLIST 21-13 **EAR IRRIGATIONS**

Steps	S	U	Comments
1. Wash hands.	————	————	
2. Gather equipment and supplies.	————	————	
3. Explain procedure to client.	————	————	
4. Position client in side-lying position with ear to be treated uppermost.	————	————	
5. If cerumen occludes outermost part of ear canal, wipe it out gently with cotton-tipped applicator.	————	————	
6. Place towel under client's head and ask client to hold irrigating basin just below tragus of ear being irrigated.	————	————	
7. Have client tilt head slightly forward toward basin.	————	————	
8. Straighten ear canal by pulling pinna down and back (children) or up and back (adults).	————	————	
9. Slowly instill irrigating solution with tip of syringe 1 cm above opening to ear canal, allowing fluid to drain out during irrigation.	————	————	
10. Dry ear and assist client to comfortable position.	————	————	
11. Dispose of supplies. Wash hands.	————	————	
12. Correctly chart medication.	————	————	

Student _____ Date _____

Instructor _____ Date _____

PERFORMANCE CHECKLIST 34-1 **TEPID SPONGING**

Steps	S	U	Comments
1. Assess temperature and pulse.	————	————	
2. Explain purpose and procedure to client.	————	————	
3. Prepare needed equipment and supplies.	————	————	
4. Wash hands. (Apply gloves if indicated).	————	————	
5. Place waterproof pads under client and remove gown.	————	————	
6. Keep bath blanket over body parts not to be sponged.	————	————	
7. Close doors and windows to prevent drafts.	————	————	
8. Check water temperature; add ethyl alcohol (optional).	————	————	
9. Immerse washcloths in water and apply wet cloths under each axilla and over groin area; if using tub, immerse client for 20 to 30 minutes.	————	————	
10. Gently sponge extremity for 5 minutes, noting response; opposite extremity may be covered by cool washcloth. In tub, squeeze water over chest and back.	————	————	
11. Dry extremity and reassess pulse, temperature, and responses.	————	————	
12. Sponge other extremities, back, and buttocks for 3 to 5 minutes each.	————	————	
13. Reassess pulse and temperature every 15 minutes.	————	————	
14. Change water and reapply sponges to axilla and groin as needed.	————	————	
15. Discontinue when body temperature falls to just above normal.	————	————	
16. Dry extremities and body parts and cover client with light bath blanket or sheet.	————	————	
17. Dispose of equipment and change bed linen if necessary. Wash hands.	————	————	
18. Measure body temperature and pulse.	————	————	
19. Record time procedure was started and terminated, vital sign changes, and response.	————	————	

Student _____ Date _____

Instructor _____ Date _____

PERFORMANCE CHECKLIST 34-2 BATHING A CLIENT

Steps	S	U	Comments
1. Assess bathing preferences.	_____	_____	
2. Review orders for precautions about movement and positioning.	_____	_____	
3. Explain procedure to client, assess ability to assist, and determine preferences for hygiene measures.	_____	_____	
4. Schedule use of shower or tub if necessary.	_____	_____	
5. Adjust room temperature and ventilation; close doors and windows; ensure privacy.	_____	_____	
6. Prepare needed equipment and supplies.			

Complete or partial bed bath

Steps	S	U	Comments
1. Offer bedpan or urinal.	_____	_____	
2. Wash hands. (Apply gloves if indicated).	_____	_____	
3. Lower side rail; assist client to a comfortable position, maintaining correct body alignment.	_____	_____	
4. Move client toward you. Place bed in high position.	_____	_____	
5. Place bath blanket over top sheet. Remove top sheet and fold or place in laundry bag.	_____	_____	
6. Remove gown properly; begin at uninjured side.	_____	_____	
7. Pull side rail up.	_____	_____	
8. Fill washbasin two-thirds full with water (43° to 46° C). Have client test temperature.	_____	_____	
9. Lower side rail. If allowed, remove pillow and raise head of bed 30 to 45 degrees; place bath towel under head.	_____	_____	
10. Place towel over chest.	_____	_____	
11. Form a mitt with washcloth; immerse in water and wring out.	_____	_____	
12. Wash eyes without soap, using different sections of mitt for each eye, moving from inner to outer canthus; dry eyes thoroughly.	_____	_____	
13. Ask client if soap is preferred on face; wash, rinse, and dry forehead, cheeks, nose, neck, and ears.	_____	_____	
14. Allow men to shave now or after bath.	_____	_____	
15. Remove bath blanket from arm farthest from you; tuck bath towel under arm.	_____	_____	
16. Wash arm with soap and water using long, frim strokes from distal to proximal areas.	_____	_____	
17. If possible, rinse arm above head to wash axilla thoroughly.	_____	_____	
18. Rinse and dry arm and axilla; apply deodorant or talcum powder if used.	_____	_____	
19. Fold bath towel in half and lay it on bed near client. Place basin on towel.	_____	_____	
20. Immerse client's hand in water; soak 3 to 5 minutes.	_____	_____	
21. Wash hand and fingernails, remove basin, and dry hand.	_____	_____	
22. Repeat steps 16 to 21 for other arm and hand.	_____	_____	
23. Check temperature of water and change if necessary.	_____	_____	
24. Cover chest with towel and fold bath blanket down to umbilicus.			

25. With one hand, lift edge of towel from chest. With mitted hand, bathe chest. Take care to wash skinfolds under female client's breasts. Dry.

26. Place bath towel lengthwise over chest and abdomen and fold blanket down to pubic region.

27. Hold bath towel with one hand; wash abdomen with mitted hand, giving special attention to umbilicus and abdominal folds. Dry.

28. Apply clean gown or pajama top.

29. Cover chest and abdomen with bath towel; expose far leg by folding back bath blanket, keeping perineum draped.

30. Bend knee with one arm beneath client's leg; raise leg to slide bath towel underneath.

31. Place basin on towel near client's foot; place foot in basin to soak while washing leg.

32. Wash from ankle to knee and knee to thigh, using long, smooth, firm strokes. Dry.

33. Cleanse foot and between toes; clean and trim nails as needed. Dry; apply lotion if needed.

34. Repeat steps 30 to 33 for other foot and leg.

35. Cover client with bath blanket; raise side rail; change bath water.

36. Lower side rail; assist client to a prone or side-lying position. Place towel beside client; slide bath blanket over shoulders and thighs.

37. Apply disposable gloves (if not done in step 2).

38. Wash, rinse, and dry back from neck to buttocks.

39. Change water and washcloth.

40. Assist client to supine or side-lying position; cover chest and arms with towel and legs with bath blanket. Avoid unnecessary exposure.

41. Wash, rinse, and dry perineal area.

42. Dispose of gloves.

43. Apply body lotion or oil as desired.

44. Assist client in dressing.

45. Comb hair; allow women to apply makeup if desired.

46. Make bed.

47. Remove soiled linen, clean and replace bathing equipment, and replace client's posessions and call light.

48. Wash hands.

Tub bath or shower

1. Clean tub or shower if necessary according to agency policy.

2. Place rubber mat in tub or shower and bathmat on floor outside.

3. Place equipment and supplies within easy reach.

4. Assist client to bathroom if necessary; ensure client wears robe and slippers.

5. Show client how to use call signal for assistance.

6. Place "occupied" sign on bathroom door.

7. Fill tub halfway with warm water (43°C); ask client to test temperature. Adjust if necessary or turn shower on and adjust temperature for client.

8. Instruct client to use safety bars when entering and leaving tub or shower.

9. Caution against use of bath oil.

10. Instruct client not to remain in tub longer than 20 minutes.

11. Check on client every 5 minutes.

12. Return to bathroom when client signals; knock before entering.   ———————   ———————

13. If client is unsteady, drain tub before client attempts to get out.   ———————   ———————

14. Assist client out of tub or shower if necessary.   ———————   ———————

15. Assist as necessary with drying.   ———————   ———————

16. Assist client as needed with donning clean gown or pajamas, slippers, and robe.   ———————   ———————

17. Assist client in returning to comfortable position in bed or chair.   ———————   ———————

18. Clean tub or shower according to agency policy; properly dispose of soiled linen and disposable equipment. Place "unoccupied" sign on door; return supplies to storage room.   ———————   ———————

19. Wash hands.   ———————   ———————

Evaluation

1. Observe client and ask if he or she feels fatigued or uncomfortable.   ———————   ———————

2. Assess skin areas that were previously soiled or reddened or showed signs of breakdown.   ———————   ———————

3. Record response to type of bath, condition of skin, and level of assistance required.   ———————   ———————

Student _____ Date _____

Instructor _____ Date _____

PERFORMANCE CHECKLIST 34-3 **PERINEAL CARE**

Steps	S	U	Comments
1. Identify clients at risk for infection.	————	————	
2. Explain procedure and purpose to client.	————	————	
3. Prepare needed equipment and supplies.	————	————	
4. Assemble supplies at bedside.	————	————	
5. Wash hands.	————	————	
6. Provide privacy.	————	————	
7. Raise bed to comfortable working position.	————	————	
8. Lower side rail and assist client to a dorsal recumbent (female) or supine (male) position.	————	————	
9. Apply gloves.	————	————	
10. Position waterproof pad or bedpan under buttocks.	————	————	
11. Fold top bed linen down; raise client's gown above genital area.	————	————	
12. Drape client with one corner of bath blanket between legs, one corner over chest, and one corner at each side of bed. Tuck corners around legs and under hips.	————	————	
13. Raise side rail.	————	————	
14. Fill washbasin with warm water (41° to 43°C).	————	————	
15. Place washbasin and tissue on overbed table; place washcloths in basin.	————	————	
16. **Female perineal care**			
a. Lower side rail and help client flex knees and spread legs.	————	————	
b. Lift lower corner of bath blanket from between legs and fold over abdomen.	————	————	
c. Wash and dry client's upper thighs.	————	————	
d. Using nondominant hand, retract labia from thigh; with dominant hand, wash carefully in skinfolds, wiping from perineum to rectum.	————	————	
e. Repeat on opposite side, using separate section of washcloth.	————	————	
f. Rinse and dry area thoroughly.	————	————	
g. Separate labia with nondominant hand; with dominant hand, wash downward from pubic area to rectum in smooth stroke, using separate section of washcloth with each stroke.	————	————	
h. If bedpan is in place, pour warm water over perineal area. Dry thoroughly.	————	————	
i. Draw lower corner of bath blanket between legs over perineum.	————	————	
j. Lower legs and assist client to side-lying position for anal care.	————	————	
17. **Male perineal care**			
a. Lower side rail.	————	————	
b. Gently place corner of bath blanket under penis.	————	————	
c. If client is uncircumcised, retract foreskin; wash urethral meatus, cleaning outward in circular motion.	————	————	
d. Discard washcloth; repeat with clean cloth until penis is clean. Rinse and dry gently.	————	————	

    e. Return foreskin to natural position.   _____   _____

    f. Wash shaft of penis with gentle but firm down-   _____   _____
        ward strokes. Rinse and dry thoroughly.

    g. Instruct client to spread legs slightly apart and   _____   _____
        gently cleanse scrotum, lifting carefully to
        wash underlying skinfolds. Rinse and dry.

    h. Fold bath blanket over perineum and assist client   _____   _____
        to side-lying position.

18. **Anal care**

    a. Wipe off excess fecal material; wash by wiping   _____   _____
        from genitalia to anus with one stroke.

    b. Discard washcloth and repeat with clean cloth un-   _____   _____
        til skin is clean. Rinse area and dry.

    c. Remove and dispose of gloves.   _____   _____

    d. Assist client to comfortable position and cover   _____   _____
        with sheet.

    e. Remove bath blanket and dispose of soiled bed   _____   _____
        linen.

    f. Return unused equipment to storage area.   _____   _____

    g. Raise side rail and lower bed to proper height.   _____   _____

    h. Return room to normal condition.   _____   _____

    i. Wash hands.   _____   _____

19. Inspect external genitalia and surrounding skin after   _____   _____
    cleansing.

20. Record procedure and any abnormal findings.   _____   _____

Student _____ Date _____

Instructor _____ Date _____

PERFORMANCE CHECKLIST 34-4   **ADMINISTERING A BACKRUB**

Steps	S	U	Comments
1. Assess for contraindications.	_____	_____	
2. Assess pulse and blood pressure if necessary.	_____	_____	
3. Explain procedure and position to client.	_____	_____	
4. Prepare needed equipment and supplies.	_____	_____	
5. Adjust bed to high, comfortable position.	_____	_____	
6. Adjust light, temperature, and sound within room.	_____	_____	
7. Position client in prone or side-lying position with back toward you. Provide privacy.	_____	_____	
8. Expose client's back, shoulders, upper arms, and buttocks. Cover rest of body with bath blanket; lay towel along back.	_____	_____	
9. Wash hands in warm water.	_____	_____	
10. Warm lotion in hands or under warm water.	_____	_____	
11. Explain that lotion will feel cool and wet.	_____	_____	
12. Apply lotion to sacral area and stroke upward from buttocks to shoulders, over upper arms, and back to buttocks, using a continuous, firm stroke and keeping hands on skin.	_____	_____	
13. Continue for at least 3 minutes.	_____	_____	
14. Knead skin by grasping it between thumb and fingers, moving upward along one side of spine from buttocks to shoulders and nape of neck, then kneading or stroking down and repeating on other side.	_____	_____	
15. End massage with long stroking movements and tell client you are ending.	_____	_____	
16. If client is on side, have him or her turn to opposite side and massage other hip.	_____	_____	
17. Wipe excess lubricant from back with bath towel.	_____	_____	
18. Assist client in redressing if necessary.	_____	_____	
19. Help client to comfortable position and raise side rails as needed.	_____	_____	
20. Properly dispose of soiled towel.	_____	_____	
21. Wash hands.	_____	_____	
22. Ask if client feels comfortable or has any areas of pain or tension.	_____	_____	
23. Reassess pulse and blood pressure.	_____	_____	
24. Record response to massage and condition of skin.	_____	_____	

Student _____ Date _____

Instructor _____ Date _____

PERFORMANCE CHECKLIST 34-5 NAIL AND FOOT CARE

Steps	S	U	Comments
1. Identify clients at risk for foot or nail problems.	————	————	
2. Explain procedure to client.	————	————	
3. Prepare needed equipment and supplies.	————	————	
4. Obtain physician's order for cutting nails if necessary.	————	————	
5. Wash hands.	————	————	
6. Provide privacy.	————	————	
7. Assist client to bedside chair if possible.	————	————	
8. Place disposable bathmat under feet.	————	————	
9. Put call light within reach.	————	————	
10. Fill wash basin with warm water (43° to 44°C); test temperature.	————	————	
11. Put basin on mat and client's feet in basin.	————	————	
12. Adjust overbed table over client's lap.	————	————	
13. Fill emesis basin with warm water (43° to 44°C) and place basin on paper towels on overbed table.	————	————	
14. Have client put fingers in basin and place arms in comfortable position.	————	————	
15. Allow feet and fingernails to soak 10 to 20 minutes; rewarm water after 10 minutes.	————	————	
16. Clean gently under fingernails with orangestick.	————	————	
17. Remove basin and dry fingers thoroughly.	————	————	
18. Clip fingernails straight across and even with tips of fingers.	————	————	
19. Shape fingernails with emery board or nail file.	————	————	
20. Gently push cuticle back with orangestick.	————	————	
21. Move overbed table away from client.	————	————	
22. Put on disposable gloves and scrub callused area of feet with washcloth.	————	————	
23. Clean gently under toenails with orangestick.	————	————	
24. Remove feet from basin and dry thoroughly.	————	————	
25. Clean and trim toenails using same procedure as with fingernails.	————	————	
26. Apply lotion to feet and hands.	————	————	
27. Assist client back into bed and into comfortable position.	————	————	
28. Properly remove and dispose of gloves.	————	————	
29. Clean and return equipment and supplies to proper location.	————	————	
30. Dispose of soiled linen appropriately.	————	————	
31. Wash hands.	————	————	
32. Inspect nails and surrounding skin.	————	————	
33. Record procedure and observations.	————	————	

Student _____ Date _____

Instructor _____ Date _____

PERFORMANCE CHECKLIST 34-6 PERFORMING MOUTH CARE FOR THE UNCONSCIOUS OR DEBILITATED CLIENT

Steps	S	U	Comments
1. Assess for gag reflex.	_____	_____	
2. Position client in side-lying position with head turned toward dependent side.	_____	_____	
3. Explain procedure to client.	_____	_____	
4. Prepare needed equipment and supplies.	_____	_____	
5. Wash hands; apply disposable gloves.	_____	_____	
6. Place paper towels on overbed table; arrange equipment. Turn on suction machine; connect tubing to suction catheter.	_____	_____	
7. Provide privacy.	_____	_____	
8. Raise bed to highest position; lower side rail.	_____	_____	
9. Bring client close to side of bed near you. Ensure client's head is turned down, toward mattress.	_____	_____	
10. Place towel under client's face and emesis basin under chin.	_____	_____	
11. Retract upper and lower teeth with padded tongue blade.	_____	_____	
12. Clean mouth, teeth, roof of mouth, inside cheeks, tongue; rinse several times. Have second nurse suction as necessary.	_____	_____	
13. Apply petrolatum jelly to lips.	_____	_____	
14. Explain that procedure is completed.	_____	_____	
15. Remove and properly dispose of gloves.	_____	_____	
16. Reposition client comfortably, raise side rail, and return bed to original position.	_____	_____	
17. Clean and return equipment; dispose of soiled linen properly.	_____	_____	
18. Wash hands.	_____	_____	
19. Inspect oral cavity.	_____	_____	
20. Record procedure and observations.	_____	_____	

Student _____ Date _____

Instructor _____ Date _____

PERFORMANCE CHECKLIST 34-7 CLEANING DENTURES

Steps	S	U	Comments
1. Ask client how dentures feel and if there is any tenderness or irritation. Assess oral cavity and denture surfaces.	_____	_____	
2. Explain procedure to client; ask preference in hygiene measures.	_____	_____	
3. Prepare needed equipment and supplies.	_____	_____	
4. Wash hands.	_____	_____	
5. Arrange supplies on bedside table.	_____	_____	
6. Fill emesis basin half full with tepid water or place washcloth in sink and fill 1 inch deep.	_____	_____	
7. Have client remove dentures and place in emesis basin. If client is unable to remove dentures, grasp upper plate at front with thumb and index finger wrapped in gauze. Then gently lift lower denture from jaw and rotate one side downward to remove from mouth. Place dentures in emesis basin.	_____	_____	
8. Apply dentrifice to denture brush and scrub all surfaces.	_____	_____	
9. Rinse dentures thoroughly.	_____	_____	
10. Store dentures in tepid water in denture cup.	_____	_____	
11. Empty basin and add fresh, cool water.	_____	_____	
12. Gently brush gums, palate, and tongue with toothpaste on soft toothbrush.	_____	_____	
13. Have client rinse mouth thoroughly.	_____	_____	
14. Reinsert dentures if client wishes.	_____	_____	
15. Clean and store supplies.	_____	_____	
16. Wash hands.	_____	_____	
17. Ask client if dentures feel comfortable.	_____	_____	
18. Record procedure properly.	_____	_____	

Student _____ Date _____

Instructor _____ Date _____

PERFORMANCE CHECKLIST 34-8 SHAMPOOING HAIR IN BED

Steps	S	U	Comments
1. Assess for contraindications.	_____	_____	
2. Review physician's order for medicated shampoo.	_____	_____	
3. Explain procedure to client.	_____	_____	
4. Prepare needed equipment and supplies.	_____	_____	
5. Wash hands.	_____	_____	
6. Arrange equipment conveniently.	_____	_____	
7. Place waterproof pad under client's shoulders, neck, and head, with client positioned with head and shoulders at top edge of bed.	_____	_____	
8. Place plastic trough under client's head and washbasin at end of trough.	_____	_____	
9. Place a rolled towel under client's neck and bath towel across shoulders.	_____	_____	
10. Brush and comb client's hair.	_____	_____	
11. Fill pitcher with water (43° to 44°C). Check temperature.	_____	_____	
12. Have client hold face towel or washcloth over eyes.	_____	_____	
13. Pour water over hair until thoroughly wet.	_____	_____	
14. Apply small amount of shampoo and work up lather with both hands, starting at hairline and working toward back of neck.	_____	_____	
15. Massage scalp with fingertips while shampooing.	_____	_____	
16. Rinse hair until hair is free of soap.	_____	_____	
17. Repeat steps 14 to 16.	_____	_____	
18. Apply conditioner if requested and rinse hair thoroughly.	_____	_____	
19. Wrap client's head in bath towel.	_____	_____	
20. Dry client's face.	_____	_____	
21. Dry hair and scalp, using second towel as needed.	_____	_____	
22. Comb hair to remove tangles.	_____	_____	
23. Dry hair as quickly as possible.	_____	_____	
24. Assist client to comfortable position.	_____	_____	
25. Clean and return equipment to proper location.	_____	_____	
26. Appropriately dispose of soiled linen.	_____	_____	
27. Wash hands.	_____	_____	
28. Ask client how hair feels.	_____	_____	
29. Inspect condition of hair.	_____	_____	
30. Record and report procedure and observations.	_____	_____	

Student _____ Date _____

Instructor _____ Date _____

PERFORMANCE CHECKLIST 34-9 TAKING CARE OF CONTACT LENSES

Steps	S	U	Comments
1. Assess client's ability to manipulate lenses.	_____	_____	
2. After lenses are removed, inspect for corneal irritation.	_____	_____	
3. Prepare needed equipment and supplies.	_____	_____	
4. Discuss procedure with client.	_____	_____	
5. Have client assume supine or sitting position.	_____	_____	
6. **Remove soft lenses.**			
a. Wash hands.	_____	_____	
b. Place towel below client's face.	_____	_____	
c. Add sterile saline to client's eye.	_____	_____	
d. Ask client to look straight ahead.	_____	_____	
e. Using middle finger, retract lower lid.	_____	_____	
f. With pad of index finger of same hand, slide lens onto white of eye.	_____	_____	
g. Pull upper lid down with thumb of other hand and compress lens between thumb and index finger.	_____	_____	
h. Gently pinch lens and lift out.	_____	_____	
i. If lens sticks together, place it in palm and soak with sterile saline. Gently roll lens with index finger in back-and-forth motion.	_____	_____	
j. Clean and rinse lens. Place lens in proper cup of storage case.	_____	_____	
k. Repeat steps c to j for other eye. Secure cover of storage case.	_____	_____	
l. Dispose of towel and wash hands.	_____	_____	
7. **Remove rigid lenses.**			
a. Wash hands.	_____	_____	
b. Place towel just below client's face.	_____	_____	
c. Position lens properly over cornea.	_____	_____	
d. Place index finger on outer corner of client's eye and draw skin gently toward ear.	_____	_____	
e. Instruct client to blink. Do not release pressure on lid until blink is completed.	_____	_____	
f. If lens does not pop out, retract lid beyond edges of lens. Press lower lid against lower edge of lens.	_____	_____	
g. Allow both eyelids to close slightly and grasp lens.	_____	_____	
h. Cup lens in hand.	_____	_____	
i. Clean and rinse lens. Place in proper storage cup.	_____	_____	
j. Repeat steps c to i for other eye. Secure cover on storage case.	_____	_____	
k. Dispose of towel and wash hands.	_____	_____	

8. **Cleanse and disinfect contact lenses.**
   a. Wash hands. _____ _____
   b. Assemble supplies at bedside. _____ _____
   c. Place towel over work area. _____ _____
   d. Open lens container carefully. _____ _____
   e. On removal of lens from eye, apply 1 to 2 drops of daily surfactant cleaner on lens in palm of hand. _____
   f. Rub lens gently but thoroughly on both sides for 20 to 30 seconds. Use index finger (soft lenses) or little finger or cotton-tipped applicator soaked with cleaner (hard lenses) to clean inside lens. Be careful not to scratch lens. _____
   g. Holding lens over emesis basin, rinse thoroughly with rinsing solution (soft lenses) or cold tap water (hard lenses). _____ _____
   h. Place lenses in storage case and fill with recommended storage solution. _____ _____

Insert rigid lenses.
1. Wash hands with mild, noncosmetic soap. Rinse well; dry with clean, lint-free towel or paper towel. _____ _____
2. Place towel over chest. _____ _____
3. Remove right lens from storage case; attempt to lift straight up. _____ _____
4. Rinse with cold tap water. _____ _____
5. Wet lens with both sides using prescribed wetting solution. _____ _____
6. Place right lens concave side up on tip of index finger of dominant hand. _____ _____
7. Instruct client to look straight ahead. While retracting upper and lower eyelids, place lens gently over center of cornea. _____ _____
8. Ask client to close eyes briefly and avoid blinking. _____ _____
9. Be sure lens is centered properly by asking client if vision is blurred. _____ _____
10. Repeat steps 3 to 9 for left eye. _____ _____
11. Assist client to comfortable position. _____ _____
12. Discard soiled supplies. Discard solution in storage case; rinse case thoroughly and allow to air dry. _____ _____
13. Wash hands. _____ _____

Insert soft lenses.
1. Wash hands with mild, noncosmetic soap. Rinse well; dry with clean, lint-free towel or paper towel. _____ _____
2. Place towel over chest. _____ _____
3. Remove right lens from storage case and rinse with recommended solution. Inspect lens for foreign materials, tears, or other damage. _____ _____
4. Check to be sure lens is not inverted. _____ _____
5. Using middle or index finger of opposite hand, retract upper lid until iris is exposed. _____ _____
6. Use middle finger or hand holding lens to pull down lower lid. _____ _____
7. Instruct client to look straight ahead and "through" the lens and finger. Gently place lens directly on cornea. Release lens slowly, starting with lower lid. _____ _____

8. If lens is on sclera, instruct client to slowly close eye and roll it toward lens. _____ _____

9. Instruct client to blink. _____ _____

10. Be sure lens is centered properly by asking client if vision is blurred.
    a. Retract eyelids. _____ _____
    b. Locate position of lens. _____ _____
    c. Ask client to look in direction opposite of lens; with index finger, position lens over cornea. _____ _____
    d. Have client look slowly toward lens. _____ _____

11. Repeat steps 3 to 10 for other eye. _____ _____

12. Assist client to comfortable position. _____ _____

13. Discard soiled supplies. Discard solution in storage case; rinse case thoroughly and allow to air dry. _____ _____

14. Wash hands. _____ _____

15. Ask client if lenses feel comfortable. _____ _____

16. Record or report signs or symptoms of visual alterations observed during procedure. _____ _____

17. Record times of lens insertion and removal. _____ _____

Student _____ Date _____

Instructor _____ Date _____

PERFORMANCE CHECKLIST 34-10 CARE OF A BEHIND-THE-EAR HEARING AID

Steps	S	U	Comments
1. Assess client's knowledge and routine for cleansing of and caring for hearing aid.	_____	_____	
2. Determine hearing level with hearing aid.	_____	_____	
3. Explain procedure.	_____	_____	
4. Assess whether aid is working.	_____	_____	
5. Check tubing, earmold, or cerumen accumulation.	_____	_____	
6. Prepare needed equipment and supplies.	_____	_____	
7. Clean hearing aid.			
a. Wash hands.	_____	_____	
b. Assemble supplies.	_____	_____	
c. Detach earmold from battery.	_____	_____	
d. Soak earmold in warm water and soap.	_____	_____	
e. Wash ear canal; rinse and dry.	_____	_____	
f. Clean earmold hole if cerumen has built up.	_____	_____	
g. Rinse earmold with water and allow to dry.	_____	_____	
h. Clean connecting tube.	_____	_____	
i. Reconnect earmold before inserting or storing.	_____	_____	
8. Insert hearing aid.			
a. Check batteries and replace if necessary.	_____	_____	
b. Turn aid off and turn volume down.	_____	_____	
c. Place earmold in external ear canal; gently press and twist until mold feels snug.	_____	_____	
d. Bring connecting tube up and over, toward back of ear. Battery device fits around upper ear.	_____	_____	
e. Adjust volume gradually.	_____	_____	
f. Remove soiled equipment.	_____	_____	
g. Dispose of used supplies.	_____	_____	
h. Wash hands.	_____	_____	
9. Assess whether aid is working.	_____	_____	
10. Document that aid is removed and stored if client is undergoing surgery or special procedure.	_____	_____	
11. Report any communication difficulties.	_____	_____	
12. Note hearing aid on Kardex.	_____	_____	

Student _____ Date _____

Instructor _____ Date _____

PERFORMANCE CHECKLIST 34-11   **MAKING A CONVENTIONAL UNOCCUPIED BED**

Steps	S	U	Comments
1. Assess client for incontinence or excess drainage.	_____	_____	
2. Assess activity orders and mobility.	_____	_____	
3. Explain procedure and ask client to sit up in chair.	_____	_____	
4. Prepare clean linen.	_____	_____	
5. Wash hands.	_____	_____	
6. Arrange clean linen on bedside table or chair; remove unnecessary equipment.	_____	_____	
7. Lower side rail; remove call light.	_____	_____	
8. Adjust bed height to comfortable working position.	_____	_____	
9. Loosen linen, moving from head to foot; move to other side, lower side rail, and loosen linen.	_____	_____	
10. Remove and fold bedspread and blanket separately; discard in linen bag if not to be reused.	_____	_____	
11. Remove soiled pillow cases and remainder of linen properly and discard in linen bag.	_____	_____	
12. Slide mattress to head of bed.	_____	_____	
13. Wipe off any moisture on mattress; dry thoroughly.	_____	_____	
14. From side of bed where linen is placed, spread mattress pad smoothly over mattress.	_____	_____	
15. Unfold bottom sheet in half and place crease lengthwise along center of bed.	_____	_____	
16. Open sheet at center of bed.	_____	_____	
17. Smooth bottom layer of sheet across mattress on your side; allow edge to hang 25 cm over edge.	_____	_____	
18. Note that lower hem of bottom sheet should lie seam down, even witth bottom edge of mattress.	_____	_____	
19. Pull remaining top portion of sheet over top edge of mattress.	_____	_____	
20. Miter top corners of bottom sheet.			
a. Face head of bed diagonally.	_____	_____	
b. Place hand farthest from head of bed under top corner of mattress and lift.	_____	_____	
c. With other hand, tuck top edge of bottom sheet smoothly under mattress.	_____	_____	
d. Face side of bed and pick up top edge of sheet.	_____	_____	
e. Lift sheet and place on top of mattress to form triangular fold with lower base of fold even with side edge of mattress.	_____	_____	
f. Tuck lower edge of sheet under mattress.	_____	_____	
g. Hold portion of sheet covering side edge of mattress in place with one hand; with other hand, tuck top of triangular fold under mattress.	_____	_____	
21. Tuck rest of sheet under mattress.	_____	_____	
22. Unfold drawsheet in half and lay crease lengthwise along center of bed (optional).	_____	_____	
23. Open sheet at center of bed.	_____	_____	
24. Smooth bottom layer of draw sheet over mattress and tuck excess under foot of mattress.	_____	_____	
25. Spread bottom sheet smoothly over edge of mattress from head to foot of bed.	_____	_____	

26. Miter top corners of bottom sheet tautly (see step 20). Tuck remaining edges of bottom sheet under mattress. _____ _____

27. Apply waterproof pad or bath blanket over draw sheet if needed. _____ _____

28. Move to side of bed where linen is located. _____ _____

29. Place top sheet over bed with vertical center fold down middle of bed. _____ _____

30. Open sheet out from head to foot, with seam up and even with top edge of mattress. _____ _____

31. Spread excess sheet over bottom edge of mattress. _____ _____

32. Make horizontal toe pleat (optional). _____ _____

33. Tuck in remaining portion of sheet on one side of foot of mattress (optional). _____ _____

34. Place blanket on bed, unfolding so crease runs lengthwise along middle of bed. _____ _____

35. Spread blanket evenly over bed. _____ _____

36. Place spread over bed; tuck top edge of spread over and under top edge of blanket. _____ _____

37. Make a cuff by turning edge of top sheet down over top edge of blanket and spread. _____ _____

38. Standing at one side of foot of bed, tuck top sheet, blanket, and spread together under mattress. Make modified mitered corners with top sheet, blanket, and spread.
    a. Lift linens to form triangular fold and lay it on bed. _____ _____
    b. Tuck loose edge hanging down under side of mattress. _____ _____
    c. Bring triangular fold down over mattress, holding linen in place along side of mattress. _____ _____

39. Go to other side of bed. Spread sheet, blanket, and spread out evenly. Fold top edge of spread over blanket; make cuff with top sheet. Make modified mitered corner at foot of bed. _____ _____

40. Replace pillowcases and position pillows at center of head of bed. _____ _____

41. Place call light within client's reach and return bed to comfortable height. _____ _____

42. Fold back top covers to one side or fanfold down to bottom third of bed. _____ _____

43. Rearrange furniture; place personal items within reach. _____ _____

44. Discard soiled linen properly. _____ _____

45. Wash hands. _____ _____

46. Evaluate tolerance to sitting up in chair. Ask if client feels weak or dizzy; assess blood pressure if necessary. _____ _____

Student _____ Date _____

Instructor _____ Date _____

PERFORMANCE CHECKLIST 34-12 **MAKING A CONVENTIONAL OCCUPIED BED**

Steps	S	U	Comments
1. Assess client for incontinence or excess drainage.	_____	_____	
2. Check chart for orders or specific precautions for movement and positioning.	_____	_____	
3. Explain procedure and assess client's ability to move.	_____	_____	
4. Prepare clean linens.	_____	_____	
5. Wash hands.	_____	_____	
6. Arrange clean linen on bedside table.	_____	_____	
7. Remove all unnecessary equipment.	_____	_____	
8. Provide privacy.	_____	_____	
9. Lower side rail. Remove call light.	_____	_____	
10. Adjust bed height to comfortable working position.	_____	_____	
11. Loosen top linens at foot of bed.	_____	_____	
12. Remove bedspread and blanket separately and fold properly for reuse or place in linen bag.	_____	_____	
13. Cover client with bath blanket; ask client to hold top edge of blanket or tuck blanket under shoulder.	_____	_____	
14. Bring top sheet under bath blanket to foot of bed; remove and place in linen bag.	_____	_____	
15. With another nurse, slide mattress toward head of bed.	_____	_____	
16. Position client on side on far side of bed, facing away from you. Adjust pillow under head. Ensure side rail is up.	_____	_____	
17. Loosen bottom linens, moving from head to foot of bed	_____	_____	
18. Fanfold bottom sheet and draw sheet toward client, tucking edges just under buttocks, back, and shoulders. Do not fanfold mattress pad if it is to be reused.	_____	_____	
19. Wipe any moisture from mattress with towel and disinfectant.	_____	_____	
20. Apply clean linen to exposed half of bed.			
a. Place clean mattress pad on bed and fanfold top layer over mattress toward client. (Smooth reused pad over mattress.)	_____	_____	
b. Unfold bottom sheet in similar manner, fanfold it toward client, and smooth the nearer half over mattress, allowing it to hang about 25 cm over edge and even with lower edge of mattress.	_____	_____	
21. Correctly miter bottom sheet.	_____	_____	
22. Tuck remainder of sheet under mattress, moving from head to foot of bed.	_____	_____	
23. Position draw sheet so it will lie under buttocks and torso; fanfold top layer toward client, and smooth and tuck the side near you (optional).	_____	_____	
24. Place waterproof pad over draw sheet with center fold against client's side and far half fanfolded toward client.	_____	_____	
25. Raise side rail and move to other side of bed.	_____	_____	

26. Lower side rail. Assist client in rolling slowly to other side, over folds of linen. _____ _____

27. Loosen and remove soiled linen and place in linen bag. _____ _____

28. Spread clean fanfolded linen smoothly over edge of mattress from head to foot of bed. _____ _____

29. Assist client in rolling back into supine position. _____ _____

30. Reposition pillow. _____ _____

31. Miter and tuck top corner of bottom sheet. _____ _____

32. Pull bottom sheet tight and tuck excess linen under mattress. _____ _____

33. Smooth fanfolded draw sheet over bottom sheet and tuck from middle to top and then bottom. _____ _____

34. Place top sheet over client. _____ _____

35. Ask client to hold clean top sheet or tuck under shoulder while removing bath blanket; discard blanket into linen bag. _____ _____

36. Place blanket on bed, with its top edge 15 to 20 cm from sheet's top edge. _____ _____

37. Apply bedspread in similar manner. Make cuff by turning edge of top sheet down over top edge of blanket and spread. _____ _____

38. At foot of bed, tuck top linens under mattress, keeping top sheet and blanket together. Make sure linens are loose enough for client's feet. _____ _____

39. Make modified mitered corners of top linen at foot of bed to secure top linen, but do not tuck corners. _____ _____

40. Raise side rails. _____ _____

41. Change pillowcase and reposition pillow under head. _____ _____

42. Reposition call light within client's reach. _____ _____

43. Return bed to comfortable position and height. _____ _____

44. Open room curtains; rearrange furniture and personal items to original positions. _____ _____

45. Discard dirty linen appropriately. _____ _____

46. Wash hands. _____ _____

Student _____ Date _____

Instructor _____ Date _____

PERFORMANCE CHECKLIST 35-1 INSERTING A NASOGASTRIC TUBE (LARGE OR SMALL BORE) FOR ENTERAL FEEDINGS

Steps	S	U	Comments
1. Assess client's need for tube feeding and intubation.	_____	_____	
2. Assess for appropriate route of administration.	_____	_____	
3. Explain procedure to client.	_____	_____	
4. Wash hands.	_____	_____	
5. Assemble equipment at bedside.	_____	_____	
6. Stand on right side of bed if right-handed (or on left side if left-handed).	_____	_____	
7. Position client correctly.	_____	_____	
8. Place bath towel over client's chest. Keep tissue within client's reach.	_____	_____	
9. Instruct client to breathe normally, and occlude one naris at a time to select naris with greater air flow.	_____	_____	
10. Determine length of tube to be inserted and mark with tape.			
a. Traditional method: measure distance from tip of nose to earlobe to xiphoid process to sternum.	_____	_____	
b. Hanson method: mark 50 cm point on tube, then do traditional measurement. Tube insertion is midway point between 50 cm (20 inches) and traditional mark.	_____	_____	

Large-bore intubation

Steps	S	U	Comments
11. Prepare nasogastric tube for intubation.			
a. Do not ice plastic tubes.	_____	_____	
b. Curl tube around several times.	_____	_____	
12. Apply gloves.	_____	_____	
13. Lubricate nasogastric tube 10 to 20 cm.	_____	_____	
14. Alert client that insertion will begin. Gently insert tube through nostril to back of throat, aiming back and down toward ear.	_____	_____	
15. Flex head toward chest after tube has passed through nasopharynx. Allow client to relax.	_____	_____	
16. Encourage client to swallow by offering small sips of water or ice chips and advance tube as client swallows. Rotate tube 180 degrees while inserting.	_____	_____	
17. Emphasize need to mouth breathe and swallow.	_____	_____	
18. Advance tube each time client swallows until desired length is passed.	_____	_____	
19. If resistance is met or client starts to gag, choke, or become cyanotic, stop and pull tube back. Check for position of tube.	_____	_____	
20. Check placement of tube.			
a. Ask client to talk.	_____	_____	
b. Attach catheter-tipped syringe to end of nasogastric tube. Aspirate gently to obtain gastric contents.	_____	_____	
c. Measure pH of aspirate with pH paper.	_____	_____	
d. If tube is not in stomach, advance another 2.5 to 5 cm (1 to 2 inches); check position.	_____	_____	
21. Apply tincture of benzoin to tip of nose and tube. Allow to dry.	_____	_____	

22. Secure tube with tape and avoid pressure on naris. _____ _____
23. Obtain x-ray film of abdomen (tube must be radi-opaque). _____ _____

Small-bore intubation

24. Prepare tube for intubation.
    a. Do not ice plastic tubes. _____ _____
    b. Inject 10 ml of water from 30 ml syringe with Lyer-Lok tip into the tube. _____ _____
    c. Properly insert guidewire or stylet into tube. _____ _____
    d. Dip weighted tip of tube into glass of water. _____ _____
25. Apply clean gloves. _____ _____
26. Insert tube through nostril to back of throat, aiming back and down toward ear. _____ _____
27. Flex head toward chest after tube has passed through na-sopharynx. _____ _____
28. Encourage client to swallow by giving small sips of wa-ter or ice chips and advance tube as client swallows. Rotate tube 180 degrees while inserting. _____ _____
29. Emphasize need to mouth breathe and swallow. _____ _____
30. Advance tube each time client swallows until desired length is passed. _____ _____
31. If resistance is met or client starts to gag, choke, or be-come cyanotic, stop and pull tube back. Check for posi-tion. _____ _____
32. Check placement of tube.
    a. Aspirate gastric contents with syringe. _____ _____
    b. Measure pH of aspirate with pH paper. _____ _____
    c. Obtain chest x-ray film of tube placement. _____ _____
33. Apply tincture of benzoin on top of nose and tube. Al-low to dry. _____ _____
34. Secure tube with tape and avoid pressure on naris. An-chor tubing to gown if possible. _____ _____
35. Position client on right side until radiological confirma-tion of placement is verified. _____ _____
36. Leave stylet in place until placement is confirmed by x-ray film. _____ _____

After insertion

37. Remain with client. _____ _____
38. Administer oral hygiene frequently. Cleanse tubing at nostril. _____ _____
39. Remove gloves; dispose of equipment; wash hands. _____ _____
40. Record type of tube placed and tolerance. _____ _____

Student _____ Date _____

Instructor _____ Date _____

PERFORMANCE CHECKLIST 35-2 INITIATING ENTERAL TUBE FEEDINGS

Steps	S	U	Comments
1. Assess client for feedings.	_____	_____	
2. Verify physician's order.	_____	_____	
3. Place client in high-Fowler's position.	_____	_____	
4. Assemble necessary equipment.	_____	_____	
5. Wash hands and apply gloves.	_____	_____	
6. Determine placement of gastric tube.			
a. Aspirate secretions.	_____	_____	
b. Observe for abdominal distention.	_____	_____	
c. Auscultate for bowel sounds.	_____	_____	
7. Administer feeding.			
a. Bolus or intermittent feeding:			
(1) Pinch proximal end of tube.	_____	_____	
(2) Attach syringe and elevate.	_____	_____	
(3) Fill syringe with formula; allow to empty gradually.	_____	_____	
(4) If gavage bag is used, use same procedure.	_____	_____	
b. Continuous drip method:			
(1) Hang gavage bag to IV pole.	_____	_____	
(2) Connect end of bag to proximal end of feeding tube.	_____	_____	
(3) Connect infusion pump; set rate.	_____	_____	
8. Administer additional water as ordered.	_____	_____	
9. Remove and dispose of gloves. Wash hands.	_____	_____	
10. Clamp proximal end of tube when feedings are not being administered.	_____	_____	
11. Administer water via tube as ordered.	_____	_____	
12. Record amount and type.	_____	_____	

Student _____ Date _____

Instructor _____ Date _____

PERFORMANCE CHECKLIST 35-3 ADMINISTERING ENTERAL FEEDINGS VIA GASTROSTOMY OR JEJUNAL TUBE

Steps	S	U	Comments
1. Assess client's need for enteral feedings.	————	————	
2. Auscultate for bowel sounds.	————	————	
3. Verify physician's orders.	————	————	
4. Assess gastrostomy or jejunostomy site.	————	————	
5. Wash hands.	————	————	
6. Assemble equipment.	————	————	
7. Prepare bag and tubing to administer formula.	————	————	
8. Explain procedure to client.	————	————	
9. Position client.	————	————	
10. Verify placement of tube.			
a. Gastrostomy tube			
(1) Aspirate gastric secretions and check gastric residual.	————	————	
(2) Auscultate over left upper quadrant with stethoscope, and inject 10 to 20 ml of air into tube.	————	————	
b. Jejunal tube: aspirate intestinal secretions and check for residual.	————	————	
11. Initiate feeding.			
a. Gastrostomy tube			
(1) Bolus or intermittent feeding			
(a) Pinch proximal end of gastrostomy tube.	————	————	
(b) Attach syringe to end of tube and elevate to 18 inches above client's abdomen.	————	————	
(c) Fill syringe with formula. Allow syringe to empty gradually; refill until prescribed amount has been delivered to client.	————	————	
(d) If gavage bag is used, attach bag to end of feeding tube and raise bag 18 inches above client's abdomen. Fill bag with prescribed amount of formula, and allow bag to empty gradually over 30 minutes.	————	————	
(2) Continuous drip method			
(a) Hand gavage bag to IV pole.	————	————	
(b) Connect end of bag to proximal end of gastrostomy tube.	————	————	
(c) Connect infusion pump and set rate.	————	————	
(3) When tube feedings are not being administered, clamp proximal end of gastrostomy tube.	————	————	
(4) Administer water via feeding tube as ordered with or between feedings.	————	————	

      (5) Rinse bag and tubing with warm water after all
         bolus feedings. _____ _____

      (6) Advance tube feeding. _____ _____

  b. Jejunal tube

      (1) Initiate continuous tube feeding (see step 11a(2). _____ _____

      (2) Advance tube feeding. _____ _____

12. Change exit site dressing as needed. Inspect site. _____ _____

13. Dispose of supplies. Wash hands. _____ _____

14. Evaluate client's tolerance of tube feeding. _____ _____

15. Observe stoma site for skin integrity. _____ _____

16. Record amount and type of feeding. _____ _____

17. Record client's response to tube feeding, patency of tube,
and any untoward effects. _____ _____

18. Report to oncoming staff: type of feeding, status of tube,
client's tolerance, and adverse effects. _____ _____

Student _____ Date _____

Instructor _____ Date _____

PERFORMANCE CHECKLIST 37-1 **PERFORMING MASSAGE TECHNIQUES**

Steps	S	U	Comments
1. Assess client's pain, body part to be massaged, and positioning.	————	————	
2. Prepare needed supplies.	————	————	
3. Explain procedure.	————	————	
4. Wash hands.	————	————	
5. Position bed.	————	————	
6. Position body part appropriately.	————	————	
7. Drape client properly.	————	————	
8. Apply lotion to hands and rub together to warm.	————	————	
9. Massage body part at least 10 minutes.	————	————	
10. Hands			
a. Make contact with one hand, then the other.	————	————	
b. Open client's palm slowly.	————	————	
c. Massage each finger outward.	————	————	
d. Use a corkscrewlike motion to massage each finger separately.	————	————	
e. Knead each small muscle in client's fingers.	————	————	
f. Glide your hands from client's fingertips to wrists.	————	————	
g. Repeat for other hand.	————	————	
11. Arms			
a. Massage from client's wrist to forearm.	————	————	
b. Knead muscles from client's forearm to shoulder.	————	————	
c. Continue to knead biceps, deltoid, and triceps muscles.	————	————	
d. Finish with gliding strokes from wrist to shoulder.	————	————	
12. Neck			
a. Support client's neck with one hand.	————	————	
b. Massage up neck with gliding stroke with other hand.	————	————	
c. Knead muscles on one side of neck.	————	————	
d. Switch hands and sides of neck.	————	————	
e. Stretch neck with one hand at top and other at bottom.	————	————	
13. When massage is complete, allow client to relax.	————	————	
14. Wash hands.	————	————	
15. Store supplies.	————	————	
16. Record massage in nurses' notes.	————	————	
17. Return to evaluate client's comfort.	————	————	

Student _____ Date _____

Instructor _____ Date _____

PERFORMANCE CHECKLIST 38-1 PERFORMING PULSE OXIMETRY

Steps	S	U	Comments
1. Identify clients who would benefit from pulse oximetry.	————	————	
2. Assess client's respiratory status.	————	————	
3. Review client's medical record.	————	————	
4. Obtain equipment and place at bedside.	————	————	
5. Explain purpose and procedure to client and family.	————	————	
6. Wash hands.	————	————	
7. Select appropriate area to apply sensor.	————	————	
8. Prepare selected site.	————	————	
9. Instruct client to breathe normally.	————	————	
10. Attach sensor probe to finger, bridge of nose, earlobe, or toe.	————	————	
11. Attach pulse oximeter sensor to client cable.			
a. Turn machine on.	————	————	
b. Listen for audible beep.	————	————	
c. Observe waveform for bar of light.	————	————	
12. Ensure that alarms for oxygen saturation and pulse rate are turned on.	————	————	
13. Read saturation level as ordered.	————	————	
14. Document client's uses of pulse oximetry equipment and oxygen saturation.	————	————	
15. Correlate with arterial blood gas measurements if available.	————	————	
16. Report client's oxygen saturations and response to changes in therapy to oncoming shift.	————	————	

Student _____ Date _____

Instructor _____ Date _____

PERFORMANCE CHECKLIST 38-2 CARING FOR THE CLIENT WITH CHEST TUBES

Steps	S	U	Comments
1. Assess the client's respiratory status.	———	———	
2. Observe:			
a. Chest tube dressing	———	———	
b. Tubing	———	———	
c. Chest drainage system	———	———	
d. Water seal for appropriate fluctuations	———	———	
e. Bubbling in water-seal bottle or chamber	———	———	
f. Type and amount of fluid drainage	———	———	
g. Bubbling in suction-control chamber	———	———	
3. Provide two shodded hemostats for each chest tube to remain at client's bedside.	———	———	
4. Position client correcttly.	———	———	
5. Tape connection between chest and drainage tubes.	———	———	
6. Coil and secure excess tubing on mattress next to client.	———	———	
7. Adjust tubing to hang in straight line from top of mattress to drainage chamber.	———	———	
8. Strip or milk drainage tubing if ordered or indicated.	———	———	
9. Wash hands.	———	———	
10. Document status of chest tube(s) and client's physical status.	———	———	

Student _____ Date _____

Instructor _____ Date _____

PERFORMANCE CHECKLIST 38-3 **PERFORMING OROPHARYNGEAL SUCTIONING (YANKAUER CATHETERS, NASOPHARYNGEAL OR NASOTRACHEAL SUCTION, ARTIFICIAL AIRWAY)**

Steps	S	U	Comments
1. Assess for signs and symptoms indicating presence of upper airway secretions.	———	———	
2. Explain procedure to client.	———	———	
3. Prepare necessary equipment and supplies.	———	———	
4. Provide for privacy.	———	———	
5. Properly position client.	———	———	
6. Place towel or pillow under client's chin.	———	———	
7. Select proper suction pressure for client and type of suction unit.	———	———	
8. Wash hands.	———	———	
9. Yankauer catheter:			
a. Apply nonsterile gloves.	———	———	
b. Prepare suction apparatus. Fill cup with water.	———	———	
c. Check functioning of equipment by suctioning small amount of water.	———	———	
d. Remove oxygen mask, if present.	———	———	
e. Insert catheter into mouth and suction correctly.	———	———	
f. Encourage client to cough. Replace oxygen mask.	———	———	
g. Rinse catheter. Turn off suction.	———	———	
h. Reassess client's respiratory status.	———	———	
i. Remove and dispose of towel. Remove and dispose of gloves in receptacle.	———	———	
j. Reposition client.	———	———	
k. Discard water and cup.	———	———	
l. Wash, rinse, and dry basin.	———	———	
m. Place catheter in clean, dry area.	———	———	
n. Wash hands.	———	———	
10. Nasopharyngeal or nasotracheal suction:			
a. Turn suction device on and set vacuum regulator to appropriate pressure.	———	———	
b. Increase supplemental oxygen as indicated or ordered.	———	———	
c. Connect tubing to suction machine.	———	———	
d. If using suction kit, open package, drape client, open catheter package, and fill basin.	———	———	
e. Apply lubricant to sterile catheter package.	———	———	
f. Apply gloves properly.	———	———	
g. Maintain catheter sterility while connecting catheter to suction.	———	———	
h. Check functioning of equipment by suctioning small amount of water.	———	———	
i. Coat distal end of catheter with water-soluble lubricant.	———	———	
j. Remove oxygen delivery device and properly insert catheter.	———	———	
k. Apply intermittent suction, encouraging client to cough when appropriate.	———	———	
l. Rinse catheter and connecting tubing with saline.	———	———	
m. Wash hands.	———	———	

11. **Artificial airway:**
    a. Wash hands.
    b. Turn suction device on and set vacuum regulator to appropriate pressure.
    c. Connect tubing to suction machine.
    d. If using sterile suction kit, open package, drape client, open catheter package, and fill basin.
    e. Apply lubricant to sterile catheter package if indicated.
    f. Apply gloves properly.
    g. Maintain catheter sterility while connecting catheter to suction.
    h. Check functioning of equipment by suctioning small amount of water.
    i. Coat distal end of tubing with water-soluble lubricant.
    j. Expose artificial airway.
    k. Hyperinflate and/or oxygenate client as indicated.
    l. Properly insert catheter into artificial airway.
    m. Pull catheter back 1 cm when resistance is met.
    n. Apply intermittent suction, encouraging client to cough as indicated.
    o. Replace oxygen delivery device. Encourage client to deep breathe.
    p. Rinse catheter and connecting tubing with normal saline.
    q. Repeat steps *k* to *p* as needed to clear secretions, allowing adequate time between suctioning.
    r. Assess client's cardiopulmonary status between suction passes.
    s. Perform nasal and oropharyngeal suctioning when tracheobronchial tree is clear.
    t. Disconnect catheter. Discard gloves and catheter appropriately.
    u. Discard towel into proper receptacle.
    v. Reposition client.
    w. Discard saline and basin (wash and store reusable basin).
    x. Wash hands.
    y. Place unopened suction kit near bedside.
12. Prepare for next suctioning.
13. Observe client for absence of secretions.
14. Document procedure and client's presuctioning and postsuctioning respiratory status.

Student _____ Date _____

Instructor _____ Date _____

PERFORMANCE CHECKLIST 38-4 **APPLYING A NASAL CANNULA**

Steps	S	U	Comments
1. Assess client.	————	————	
2. Prepare needed equipment and supplies.	————	————	
3. Explain procedure and purpose to client and family.	————	————	
4. Wash hands.	————	————	
5. Attach nasal cannula to humidified oxygen source.	————	————	
6. Adjust oxygen flow to prescribed rate.	————	————	
7. Place tips of cannula into nares.	————	————	
8. Adjust band until cannula fits snugly and comfortably.	————	————	
9. Secure oxygen tubing to clothes.	————	————	
10. Check cannula every 8 hours.	————	————	
11. Keep humidification jar filled at all times.	————	————	
12. Assess nares and external nose for skin breakdown every 6 to 8 hours.	————	————	
13. Check oxygen flow rate and physician's orders every 8 hours.	————	————	
14. Wash hands.	————	————	
15. Inspect client for relief of symptoms.	————	————	
16. Observe nares and superior surface of ears for skin breakdown.	————	————	
17. Record procedure and observations properly.	————	————	

Student _____ Date _____

Instructor _____ Date _____

PERFORMANCE CHECKLIST 38-5 **USING HOME OXYGEN EQUIPMENT**

Steps	S	U	Comments
1. Assess client's and family's ability to use equipment.	_____	_____	
2. Assess client's or family's ability to observe for hypoxia.	_____	_____	
3. Explain procedure to client and family.	_____	_____	
4. Prepare equipment.	_____	_____	
5. Wash hands.	_____	_____	
6. Demonstrate steps for oxygen therapy.	_____	_____	
7. Prepare Liberator and Stroller for use.	_____	_____	
8. Have client or family perform each step.	_____	_____	
9. Discuss signs and symptoms of respiratory infection.	_____	_____	
10. Instruct to notify physician if signs or symptoms occur.	_____	_____	
11. Wash hands.	_____	_____	
12. Record teaching, information, and learning.	_____	_____	

Student _____ Date _____

Instructor _____ Date _____

PERFORMANCE CHECKLIST 38-6 **PERFORMING CARDIOPULMONARY RESUSCITATION**

Steps	S	U	Comments
One nurse			
1. Assess victim for unresponsiveness; palpate carotid pulse.	_____	_____	
2. Call for help.	_____	_____	
3. Place victim supine on hard surface.	_____	_____	
4. Kneel at level of victim's shoulders.	_____	_____	
5. Open victim's airway with head tilt/chin lift or jaw thrust maneuver.	_____	_____	
6. Check for airway obstruction.	_____	_____	
7. Prepare for artificial respiration by pinching nose and occluding victim's mouth (or infant's nose and mouth) with yours or by using Ambu bag.	_____	_____	
8. Properly administer artificial respiration with correct timing.	_____	_____	
9. Observe for rise and fall of chest wall; if necessary, reposition head and neck and recheck for airway obstruction.	_____	_____	
10. If suction available, suction any secretions.	_____	_____	
11. Assess for carotid pulse (or brachial pulse in infant).	_____	_____	
12. Begin external cardiac compressions on pulseless victim, using proper technique for age.	_____	_____	
13. Adult			
a. Use proper hand position, one hand on top of the other over sternum.	_____	_____	
b. Extend or interlace fingers.	_____	_____	
c. Lock elbows, keep arms straight and shoulders directly over victim's sternum, and compress chest 3.8 to 5.0 cm 80 to 100 times per minute.	_____	_____	
d. Ventilate lungs twice for artificial respiration.	_____	_____	
e. Reassess victim after four cycles.	_____	_____	
14. Infant (1 to 12 months)			
a. Use proper hand position, index finger over sternum.	_____	_____	
b. With two fingers, compress chest 1.3 to 2.5 cm at least 100 times per minute.	_____	_____	
c. Ventilate lungs at end of every fifth compression.	_____	_____	
d. Reassess victim after 10 cycles.	_____	_____	
15. Child (1 to 7 years)			
a. Use proper hand position, one hand next to other over sternum.	_____	_____	
b. Compress sternum with one hand 2.5 to 3.8 cm 80 to 100 compressions a minute.	_____	_____	
c. Ventilate lungs after every fifth compression.	_____	_____	
d. Reassess victim after 10 cycles.	_____	_____	
Two nurses			
1. Position nurse at side to perform external compression 80 to 100 times per minute.	_____	_____	
2. Other nurse remains at victim's head, maintains open airway, and monitors carotid pulse.	_____	_____	
3. Change positions when compressor is fatigued.	_____	_____	

Student _____ Date _____

Instructor _____ Date _____

PERFORMANCE CHECKLIST 39-1 **PERFORMING VENIPUNCTURE WITH AN OVER-THE-NEEDLE PLASTIC CATHETER (ONC)**

Steps	S	U	Comments
1. Assess client for fluid or electrolyte imbalances.	————	————	
2. Identify client and explain procedure.	————	————	
3. Assemble needed equipment at bedside.	————	————	
4. Identify accessible vein.	————	————	
5. Wash hands.	————	————	
6. Using aseptic technique, open sterile packages.	————	————	
7. Using "five rights" of medications; confirm correct solutions.	————	————	
8. If using bottled solution, remove metal cap and disks beneath it.	————	————	
9. Open infusion set, maintaining sterility of both ends.	————	————	
10. Place roller clamp 2 to 4 cm below drip chamber and close clamp.	————	————	
11. Insert infusion set into fluid bag.			
a. Properly remove cover from IV bag.	————	————	
b. Remove cover from spike and insert spike into opening of bag or into rubber stopper of bottle.	————	————	
12. Fill infusion tubing.			
a. Compress drip chamber and release.	————	————	
b. Remove needle protector and open roller clamp for fluid to travel from drip chamber to needle adapter.	————	————	
c. Close roller clamp after tube is filled.	————	————	
d. Check tubing for air bubbles.	————	————	
e. Replace needle protector.	————	————	
13. Select appropriate IV needle or ONC.	————	————	
14. Select distal site of vein to be used.	————	————	
15. If necessary, clip body hair at insertion site.	————	————	
16. If possible, place extremity in dependent position.	————	————	
17. Place tourniquet 10 to 12 cm above site; check distal pulse.	————	————	
18. Choose well-dilated vein. If necessary, use methods to foster vein dilation.	————	————	
19. Apply disposable gloves.	————	————	
20. Properly cleanse insertion site.	————	————	
21. Perform venipuncture.			
a. Butterfly needle: insert needle at 20- to 30-degree angle, with bevel 1 cm distal to actual site.	————	————	
b. ONC: insert bevel at 20- to 30-degree angle, distal to actual site.	————	————	
22. Confirm that vein has been entered by blood flow through needle or catheter tubing.	————	————	
23. Advance catheter ¼ inch into vein and loosen stylet; continue advancing until hub rests at site.	————	————	
24. Maintaining sterility, connect adapter of infusion set to hub of ONC or needle.	————	————	
25. Stabilize catheter and release tourniquet.	————	————	

26. Release roller clamp to begin infusion. _____ _____
27. Apply povidone-iodine solution or ointment at venipuncture site. _____ _____
28. Secure catheter or needle.
   a. Place strip of tape under catheter and cross it over catheter. _____ _____
   b. Place second strip directly across catheter. _____ _____
   c. Place third strip under needle adapter and cross tape over infusion tubing. _____ _____
   d. Place 2 × 2 gauze over catheter and secure with tape. _____ _____
   e. Secure tubing to catheter with tape. _____ _____
29. Record date and time of procedure and nurse's initials and title on dressing. _____ _____
30. Adjust flow rate. _____ _____
31. Discard gloves and supplies. Wash hands. _____ _____
32. Observe response to procedure. _____ _____
33. Record procedure and observations. _____ _____

Student _____ Date _____

Instructor _____ Date _____

PERFORMANCE CHECKLIST 39-2 REGULATING INTRAVENOUS FLOW RATES

Steps	S	U	Comments
1. Observe patency of IV line and needle.	_____	_____	
2. Check medical record for correct solution and additives.	_____	_____	
3. Know calibration of infusion set.	_____	_____	
4. Select proper formula to calculate flow.	_____	_____	
5. Place infusion pump or volume control device at bedside, if ordered.	_____	_____	
6. Maintain "five rights" of drug administration.	_____	_____	
7. Calculate hourly rate by dividing volume by hours.	_____	_____	
8. Place adhesive tape on IV bottle or bag next to volume markings.	_____	_____	
9. Using correct formula, calculate minute rate based on drop factor of infusion set used.	_____	_____	
10. Time flow rate by counting drops in drip chamber for 1 minute with watch.	_____	_____	
11. Adjust roller clamp as needed.	_____	_____	
12. For infusion pump:			
a. Place electronic eye on drip chamber.	_____	_____	
b. Place infusion tubing within control box.	_____	_____	
c. Start mechanism.	_____	_____	
d. Monitor infusion rates hourly.	_____	_____	
e. Assess patency of IV system if alarm sounds.	_____	_____	
13. For volume control device:			
a. Place device between IV bag and insertion spike of infusion set.	_____	_____	
b. Place correct amount of fluid in device.	_____	_____	
c. Assess system hourly; add fluid and regulate flow rate as appropriate.	_____	_____	
14. Observe response to procedure and assess IV site.	_____	_____	
15. Record procedure and observations.	_____	_____	

Student _____ Date _____

Instructor _____ Date _____

PERFORMANCE CHECKLIST 39-3 CHANGING IV SOLUTIONS AND TUBING

Steps	S	U	Comments
Changing IV solution	_____	_____	
1. Assess physician's orders; have IV solution prepared at least 1 hour before needed. Be sure it has been delivered to floor; check for correct solution and proper labeling.			
2. Change solution when it is in neck of bottle or bag.	_____	_____	
3. Be sure drip chamber is half full.	_____	_____	
4. Wash hands.	_____	_____	
5. Prepare new solution for changing by removing cover from entry site of plastic bag or removing cap and metal and rubber disks from glass bottle. Maintain sterility of container entry site.	_____	_____	
6. Adjust roller clamp to reduce flow rate.	_____	_____	
7. Remove old solution from IV pole.	_____	_____	
8. Quickly remove spike from old IV solution and, without touching its tip, spike new solution container.	_____	_____	
9. Hang new solution.	_____	_____	
10. Check for air in tubing.	_____	_____	
11. Make sure drip chamber contains solution.	_____	_____	
12. Adjust flow rate to prescribed rate.	_____	_____	
13. Observe IV system for patency.	_____	_____	
14. Observe for complications and response to therapy.	_____	_____	
Changing IV tubing			
15. Determine when new infusion set is needed.	_____	_____	
16. Assemble needed supplies.	_____	_____	
17. Explain procedure to client.	_____	_____	
18. Wash hands.	_____	_____	
19. Open new infusion set, keeping protective cover in place.	_____	_____	
20. Place sterile 2 × 2 or 4 × 4 gauze near puncture site.	_____	_____	
21. Remove IV dressing if necessary to see needle or catheter hub.	_____	_____	
22. Take new tubing and move roller clamp to "off" position.	_____	_____	
23. Regulate drip rate on old tubing to slow infusion.	_____	_____	
24. With old tubing in place, compress drip and fill chambers.	_____	_____	
25. Discontinue old tubing from solution and hang drip chamber over IV pole.	_____	_____	
26. Place insertion spike of new tubing into old solution opening; hang solution on IV pole.	_____	_____	
27. Compress and release drip chamber on new tubing.	_____	_____	
28. Open roller clamp; remove protective cap from needle adapter; flush tubing with solution.	_____	_____	

29. Place needle adapter of new tubing, cap off, between gauze near puncture site.   _____   _____

30. Turn roller clamp on old tubing to "off."   _____   _____

31. Stabilize hub of IV catheter or needle and gently pull out old tubing; maintain stability while quickly inserting needle adapter of new tubing into hub.   _____   _____

32. Open roller clamp on new tubing.   _____   _____

33. Regulate drip and monitor rate hourly.   _____   _____

34. Apply new dressing if necessary.   _____   _____

35. Discard old tubing properly.   _____   _____

36. Wash hands.   _____   _____

37. Evaluate flow rate and observe for leakage.   _____   _____

38. Record procedure.   _____   _____

39. Write time and date of change on tape placed below drip chamber.   _____   _____

Student _____ Date _____

Instructor _____ Date _____

PERFORMANCE CHECKLIST 39-4 CHANGING AN IV DRESSING

Steps	S	U	Comments
1. Determine last change of dressing by observing dressing for moisture and intactness and IV system for proper functioning.	_____	_____	
2. Prepare needed equipment.	_____	_____	
3. Explain procedure to client.	_____	_____	
4. Wash hands.	_____	_____	
5. Apply disposable gloves.	_____	_____	
6. Remove old tape and gauze one piece at a time, leaving in place tape that secures needle or catheter.	_____	_____	
7. Discontinue infusion if appropriate.			
a. Turn roller clamp to "off."	_____	_____	
b. Place gauze or alcohol pad over puncture site and remove catheter or needle.	_____	_____	
c. Apply pressure to site for 1 to 2 minutes.	_____	_____	
8. Stabilizing needle or catheter with one hand, gently remove tape, securing it in place.	_____	_____	
9. Cleanse skin with adhesive remover.	_____	_____	
10. In circular motion, cleanse insertion site with povidone-iodine solution, then allow to dry.	_____	_____	
11. Replace tape to anchor catheter or needle.	_____	_____	
12. Place povidone-iodine ointment or solution on venipuncture site. Allow to dry. Place piece of narrow tape across catheter.	_____	_____	
13. Place 2 × 2 gauze or transparent dressing over puncture site.	_____	_____	
14. Reapply tape to secure needle or catheter.	_____	_____	
15. Write date and time of change on dressing.	_____	_____	
16. Discard equipment, remove and dispose of gloves, and wash hands.	_____	_____	
17. Reassess functioning of IV system.	_____	_____	
18. Record procedure and observations.	_____	_____	

Student _____ Date _____

Instructor _____ Date _____

PERFORMANCE CHECKLIST 39-5 **ADMINISTERING A BLOOD TRANSFUSION**

Steps	S	U	Comments
1. Explain procedure to client and ask about previous transfusions and reactions.	_____	_____	
2. Ask client to report symptoms during or after transfusion: headache, itching, or rash.	_____	_____	
3. Wash hands; apply disposable gloves.	_____	_____	
4. Ensure client has signed consent form.	_____	_____	
5. Establish IV line with #18- or #19-gauge catheter.	_____	_____	
6. Prepare infusion tubing with in-line filter, using Y-type administration set.	_____	_____	
7. Hang solution of 0.9% normal saline to be administered after the blood transfusion.	_____	_____	
8. Obtain blood product from blood bank, following agency protocol.	_____	_____	
9. With another nurse, confirm blood product and check client's identification.			
a. Check compatibility tag and other information on the blood bag.	_____	_____	
b. With whole blood, check ABO group and Rh type on client's chart.	_____	_____	
c. Confirm blood product against physician's order.	_____	_____	
d. Ask client's name and check armband.	_____	_____	
10. Check expiration date on blood bag.	_____	_____	
11. Inspect blood for clots.	_____	_____	
12. Take baseline vital signs before administering infusion.	_____	_____	
13. Prime infusion line with 0.9% normal saline.	_____	_____	
14. Begin infusion slowly by first filling the in-line filter.	_____	_____	
15. Adjust infusion rate to 2 ml/min for the first 15 minutes.	_____	_____	
16. Remain with client, taking vital signs every 5 minutes for the first 15 minutes, observing for flushing, itching, dyspnea, hives, or rash.	_____	_____	
17. If changes in vital signs or other symptoms lead you to suspect a reaction, *stop* the transfusion and notify the physician and blood bank.	_____	_____	
18. If no reaction is noted, maintain prescribed infusion rate, using infusion pump if necessary.	_____	_____	
19. Remain with client and observe for adverse reactions.	_____	_____	
20. Correctly record time and infusion rate, blood or blood product administered, and response.	_____	_____	
21. When infusion is completed, return blood bag and tubing to blood bank.	_____	_____	

Student _____ Date _____

Instructor _____ Date _____

PERFORMANCE CHECKLIST 39-6 **PERFORMING AN ARTERIAL PUNCTURE**

Steps	S	U	Comments
1. Explain procedure to client.	____	____	
2. Palpate radial artery.	____	____	
3. Hyperextend client's wrist over a rolled towel.	____	____	
4. Cleanse site with a circular motion using povidone-iodine and then an alcohol wipe.	____	____	
5. Apply a local anesthetic such as Xylocaine 2%.	____	____	
6. Flush 3 ml syringe with 0.5 ml of 1000 μ/ml heparin solution; empty syringe, leaving heparin in needle.	____	____	
7. Stabilize artery with nondominant hand and insert needle at an angle.	____	____	
8. Observe for pulsating flow of blood into syringe.	____	____	
9. Withdraw 2 ml blood.	____	____	
10. Remove needle from artery; expel any air in syringe, and cork syringe with an air lock.	____	____	
11. Rotate syringe to mix blood with heparin.	____	____	
12. Submerge syringe in crushed ice.	____	____	
13. Label the specimen with client's name, body temperature, and (for clients receiving oxygen therapy) inspired oxygen concentration.	____	____	
14. Transport specimens to laboratory immediately.	____	____	
15. Apply pressure to puncture site with a 2 × 2 gauze held in place for 5 minutes; hold longer for clients receiving anticoagulant therapy.	____	____	
16. Apply tape over gauze if bleeding stops.	____	____	
17. Discard equipment, dispose of gloves, and wash hands.	____	____	
18. Record times of procedure and extremity used.	____	____	

Student _____ Date _____

Instructor _____ Date _____

PERFORMANCE CHECKLIST 40-1 **COLLECTING A MIDSTREAM (CLEAN-VOIDED) SPECIMEN**

Steps	S	U	Comments
1. Assess client's ability to use toilet facilities.	——	——	
2. Prepare equipment and supplies.	——	——	
3. Explain procedure to client.	——	——	
4. Provide fluids ½ hour before collecting specimen.	——	——	
5. Wash hands.	——	——	
6. Provide privacy.	——	——	
7. Have client cleanse perineal area or assist as needed.	——	——	
8. Apply gloves.	——	——	
9. Open sterile kit.	——	——	
10. Open specimen container.	——	——	
11. Assist or allow client to cleanse perineal area and collect specimen.			
a. Male			
1. Cleanse penis and rinse.	——	——	
2. After client initiates urine, pass container into stream and collect 30 to 60 ml.	——	——	
b. Female			
1. Cleanse perineal area and rinse.	——	——	
2. After client initiates stream, pass container into stream and collect 30 to 60 ml.	——	——	
12. Remove container before urine flow stops.	——	——	
13. Place cap on container.	——	——	
14. Cleanse urine from container.	——	——	
15. Place container in plastic specimen bag.	——	——	
16. Remove bedpan (if applicable) and assist client to comfortable position.	——	——	
17. Label specimen and attach laboratory requisition slip.	——	——	
18. Remove and dispose of gloves.	——	——	
19. Wash hands.	——	——	
20. Take specimen to laboratory within 15 minutes or refrigerate.	——	——	
21. Record date and time of specimen.	——	——	

Student _____ Date _____

Instructor _____ Date _____

PERFORMANCE CHECKLIST 40-2 **INSERTING A STRAIGHT OR INDWELLING CATHETER**

Steps	S	U	Comments
1. Assess client's status.	———	———	
2. Prepare equipment and supplies.	———	———	
3. Explain procedure to client.	———	———	
4. Arrange for nursing personnel to assist if needed.	———	———	
5. Wash hands.	———	———	
6. Raise bed to comfortable working height.	———	———	
7. Stand on left side of bed if right-handed, or vice versa.	———	———	
8. Raise side rail on opposite side of bed.	———	———	
9. Provide privacy.	———	———	
10. Place waterproof pad under client.	———	———	
11. Position client.			
a. For female client, assist to dorsal recumbent position and externally rotate thighs, or position in side-lying position.	———	———	
b. For male client, assist to supine position with thighs slightly abducted.	———	———	
12. Drape client.			
a. Drape female client with bath blanket; a corner at neck, a corner over perineum, and one corner over each arm and side.	———	———	
b. Drape male client's trunk with blanket and cover lower extremities with bedsheet, exposing only genitalia.	———	———	
13. Wash perineal area with soap and water as needed and dry.	———	———	
14. With indwelling catheter, open drainage system; place drainage bag over edge of bottom bed frame and bring tube up between side rail and mattress.	———	———	
15. Position lamp to view perineal area.	———	———	
16. Open catheterization kit according to directions, maintaining sterility.	———	———	
17. Apply gloves.	———	———	
18. Organize supplies properly on sterile field.	———	———	
19. Apply sterile drape.			
a. Female: form cuff over both hands with top edge of drape. Place drape on bed between thighs, slipping cuffed edge under buttocks. Pick up fenestrated sterile drape and allow to unfold; apply over perineum, exposing labia.	———	———	
b. Male: apply sterile drape over thighs below penis. Pick up fenestrated sterile drape; allow to unfold; apply over penis with slit resting over penis.	———	———	
20. Place sterile tray on sterile drape between thighs.	———	———	
21. Open antiseptic packet and pour contents over sterile cotton balls or gauze.	———	———	
22. Open urine specimen container, keeping top sterile.	———	———	
23. Apply lubricant (2.5 to 5 cm for females and 2.5 to 7.5 cm for males) to bottom of catheter tip.	———	———	
24. Cleanse female urethral meatus.			
a. With nondominant hand, retract labia; keep hand in this position during procedure.	———	———	
b. With dominant hand, clean perineal area with cotton ball or gauze held in forceps, wiping from clitoris toward anus; use new cotton ball with each wipe.	———	———	

25. Cleanse male urethral meatus.
    a. With nondominant hand, retract foreskin of uncircumcised male; grasp penis at shaft just below glans.
    b. Retract urethral meatus; keep nondominant hand in this position throughout procedure.
    c. With dominant hand, clean penis with cotton ball or gauze held in forceps, wiping from meatus to base of glans in circular motion; repeat cleansing twice with clean cotton balls.
26. Pick up catheter about 5 to 7.5 cm from tip with dominant hand; hold end of catheter loosely coiled in palm of dominant hand.
27. Insert catheter in female client.
    a. Ask client to take deep breath, then slowly insert catheter tip through meatus.
    b. Advance catheter 5 to 7.5 cm in adult or 2.5 cm in child, or until urine flows out end; when urine appears, advance catheter another 1.2 cm.
    c. Release labia and hold catheter securely in nondominant hand.
28. Insert catheter in male client.
    a. Lift penis to position perpendicular to body and apply light traction.
    b. Ask client to bear down gently. Then slowly insert catheter tip through meatus.
    c. Advance catheter 17.5 to 20 cm in adult, 4 to 7.5 cm in child, or until urine flows out end; withdraw catheter if resistance is felt.
    d. When urine appears, advance catheter another 1.2 cm.
29. Collect urine specimen. Fill specimen cup or jar to desired level.
30. Pinch catheter with dominant hand to stop flow to move catheter end to collection tray and drain remaining urine.
31. Cover specimen cup or jar and set aside for labeling.
32. Allow bladder to empty fully or follow agency policy.
33. Remove straight, single-use catheter by withdrawing catheter slowly but smoothly.
34. Inflate balloon of indwelling catheter.
    a. Hold catheter with nondominant hand.
    b. With dominant hand, attach syringe to injection port at end of catheter.
    c. Slowly inject solution. (If client feels pain, aspirate solution back and advance catheter farther.)
    d. After balloon inflation, release catheter and pull gently to feel resistance.
35. Attach end of catheter to collecting tube.
36. Tape catheter.
    a. For female client, tape catheter to top of thigh.
    b. For male client, tape catheter to top of thigh or lower abdomen, with penis pointed toward chest.
37. Ensure no kinks or obstructions in tubing; fasten excess tubing to bottom sheet.
38. Remove gloves; dispose of equipment, drapes, and urine.
39. Assist client to comfortable position.
40. Wash and dry perineal area as needed.
41. Instruct client how to lie in bed with catheter; caution against pulling on it.
42. Wash hands.
43. Palpate bladder and ask if client is uncomfortable.
44. Observe character and amount of urine drained.
45. Record procedure and observations.

Student _____ Date _____

Instructor _____ Date _____

PERFORMANCE CHECKLIST 40-3 **PROVIDING INDWELLING CATHETER CARE**

Steps	S	U	Comments
1. Assess for bowel incontinence or discomfort at catheter insertion site.	_____	_____	
2. Prepare equipment and supplies.	_____	_____	
3. Explain procedure.	_____	_____	
4. Provide privacy.	_____	_____	
5. Wash hands.	_____	_____	
6. Position client properly.	_____	_____	
7. Place waterproof pad under client.	_____	_____	
8. Drape client.	_____	_____	
9. Apply gloves.	_____	_____	
10. Undo anchor tapes to free catheter tubing.	_____	_____	
11. Assess urethral meatus.	_____	_____	
12. Cleanse perineal tissues.			
a. Female: cleanse each labum majus; repeat to clean labia minora.	_____	_____	
b. Male: cleanse around catheter, then meatus and glans.	_____	_____	
13. Reassess meatus for discharge.	_____	_____	
14. Wipe approximately 10 cm (4-inch) length of catheter with soap and water.	_____	_____	
15. Apply ointment at meatus and along catheter.	_____	_____	
16. Dispose of supplies and gloves.	_____	_____	
17. Record and report client's condition.	_____	_____	

Student _____ Date _____

Instructor _____ Date _____

PERFORMANCE CHECKLIST 40-4 APPLYING A CONDOM CATHETER

Steps	S	U	Comments
1. Assess client's status and condition of penis.	————	————	
2. Prepare needed equipment and supplies.	————	————	
3. Explain procedure to client.	————	————	
4. Wash hands.	————	————	
5. Provide privacy.	————	————	
6. Assist client to supine position.	————	————	
7. Drape torso with bath blanket and cover lower extremities with bedsheet, exposing only genitalia.	————	————	
8. Apply gloves.	————	————	
9. Wash perineal area with soap and water and dry.	————	————	
10. Prepare drainage bag by attaching it to bed frame, and bring tubing up through side rails onto bed.	————	————	
11. Grasp penis firmly along shaft with nondominant hand.	————	————	
12. With dominant hand, hold condom sheath at tip of penis and smoothly roll sheath onto penis.	————	————	
13. Allow 2.5 to 5 cm space above end of condom catheter.	————	————	
14. Encircle penile shaft with strip of Velcro or adhesive, ensuring strip touches only condom sheath; apply snugly but not tightly.	————	————	
15. Connect drainage tubing to end of condom catheter.	————	————	
16. Fasten excess tubing to bottom sheet with clip or other device.	————	————	
17. Assist client to comfortable position.	————	————	
18. Dispose of contaminated supplies.	————	————	
19. Wash hands.	————	————	
20. Observe urinary drainage.	————	————	
21. Inspect skin on penile shaft.	————	————	
22. Record procedure and observations.	————	————	

Student _____ Date _____

Instructor _____ Date _____

PERFORMANCE CHECKLIST 40-5 PERFORMING CLOSED AND OPEN CATHETER IRRIGATION

Steps	S	U	Comments
1. Assess urine amount and type of catheter.	———	———	
2. Collect equipment and supplies.	———	———	
3. Explain procedure to client.	———	———	
4. Wash hands.	———	———	
5. Provide privacy.	———	———	
6. Position client properly.	———	———	
7. Assess for bladder distention.	———	———	
8. Closed intermittent irrigation:			
a. Prepare solution and draw into syringe.	———	———	
b. Clamp indwelling catheter below injection port.	———	———	
c. Cleanse port with swab.	———	———	
d. Insert syringe at 30-degree angle.	———	———	
e. Slowly inject fluid into catheter and bladder.	———	———	
f. Withdraw syringe, remove clamp, and allow solution to drain into bag.	———	———	
9. Closed continuous irrigation:			
a. Insert tip of irrigation tubing into bag containing solution.	———	———	
b. Close clamp on tubing and hang solution on IV pole.	———	———	
c. Open clamp, allow solution to flow through tubing, and close clamp.	———	———	
d. Connect to irrigation tubing, using triple-lumen catheter or a Y connector to double-lumen catheter.	———	———	
e. For intermittent flow, clamp tubing on drainage, open irrigation tubing, allow prescribed amount to enter bladder, close irrigation clamp, then open drainage clamp.	———	———	
10. Open irrigation:			
a. Prepare supplies.	———	———	
b. Apply gloves.	———	———	
c. Position waterproof drape.	———	———	
d. Move collection basin close to client's thigh.	———	———	
e. Disconnect catheter from tubing, allow urine to flow into basin, and cover open end of tubing with sterile cap.	———	———	
f. Insert syringe, gently instill solution, then withdraw.	———	———	
g. Allow solution to drain into basin.	———	———	
h. Repeat until drainage is clear.	———	———	
i. Once irrigation is complete, reestablish closed drainage system.	———	———	
11. Reanchor catheter to client.	———	———	
12. Dispose of supplies.	———	———	
13. Wash hands.	———	———	
14. Record type and amount of irrigation and character of drainage.	———	———	

Student _____ Date _____

Instructor _____ Date _____

PERFORMANCE CHECKLIST 41-1 **MEASURING OCCULT BLOOD IN STOOL**

Steps	S	U	Comments
1. Assess client's medical history and medications.	_____	_____	
2. Check physician's orders.	_____	_____	
3. Prepare needed equipment and supplies.	_____	_____	
4. Explain test to client.	_____	_____	
5. Be sure dietary or medication restrictions were followed.	_____	_____	
6. Wash hands.	_____	_____	
7. Apply gloves.	_____	_____	
8. Obtain uncontaminated stool specimen.	_____	_____	
9. Use tip of applicator to obtain portion of feces.	_____	_____	
10. Perform Hemoccult test.			
a. Open flap of slide; apply smear of stool in first box.	_____	_____	
b. Obtain second specimen; apply to slide's second box.	_____	_____	
c. Close slide cover; turn over to reverse side; open flap and apply two drops of Hemoccult solution on each box of guaiac paper.	_____	_____	
d. After 30 to 60 seconds, read results.	_____	_____	
e. Properly dispose of test slide.	_____	_____	
11. Dispose of applicator properly.	_____	_____	
12. Wash hands.	_____	_____	
13. Note changes in guaiac paper.	_____	_____	
14. Record test results and observations.	_____	_____	

Student _____ Date _____

Instructor _____ Date _____

PERFORMANCE CHECKLIST 41-2 ADMINISTERING A CLEANSING ENEMA

Steps	S	U	Comments
1. Assess client's status and elimination history.	————	————	
2. Review physician's order.	————	————	
3. Prepare needed equipment.	————	————	
4. Identify client and explain procedure.	————	————	
5. Assemble enema bag.	————	————	
6. Wash hands.	————	————	
7. Provide privacy.	————	————	
8. Raise bed to comfortable working height and raise side rail on opposite side.	————	————	
9. Assist client to left side-lying position with right knee flexed; children may be put in dorsal recumbent position.	————	————	
10. Place waterproof pad under buttocks.	————	————	
11. Cover client with bath blanket, exposing only rectal area.	————	————	
12. Place bedpan in accessible position.	————	————	
13. Apply gloves.	————	————	
14. Administer prepackaged enema.			
a. Remove cap from rectal tip; add more jelly to prelubricated tip if needed.	————	————	
b. Separate buttocks and locate rectum. Instruct client to exhale slowly through mouth.	————	————	
c. Insert tip of bottle into rectum 7.5 to 10 cm in adult.	————	————	
d. Squeeze bottle to empty solution into rectum and colon.	————	————	
15. Administer enema using enema bag.			
a. Add warmed water or saline in correct volume to container; check temperature of solution.	————	————	
b. Raise container, release clamp, and allow solution to flow until it fills tubing.	————	————	
c. Reclamp tubing.	————	————	
d. Lubricate 3 to 4 inches of tip of rectal tube.	————	————	
e. Gently separate buttocks and locate rectum.	————	————	
f. Ask client to relax and exhale slowly through mouth.	————	————	
g. Insert tip of rectal tube slowly, pointing tip in direction of umbilicus as appropriate for client.	————	————	
h. Hold tube in rectum throughout fluid instillation.	————	————	
i. Opening regulating clamp and allow solution to flow slowly with container at client's hip level.	————	————	
j. Raise container slowly to appropriate point (30 to 45 cm) above anus.	————	————	

k. If client complains of cramping or if fluid escapes around rectal tube, lower container or clamp tubing.   _____   _____

l. Clamp tubing when solution has infused.   _____   _____

16. Place layers of toilet tissue around tube at anus and gently withdraw rectal tube.   _____   _____

17. Ask client to lie quietly in bed to retain the solution, explaining feeling of distention is normal; for infant or young child, gently hold buttocks together.   _____   _____

18. Discard or properly cleanse and put away enema container and tubing.   _____   _____

19. Remove and discard gloves.   _____   _____

20. Assist client to bathroom or position on bedpan.   _____   _____

21. Inspect character of stool and fluid.   _____   _____

22. Assist client as needed to wash anal area with warm soap and water.   _____   _____

23. Wash hands.   _____   _____

24. Record procedure and observations.   _____   _____

Student _____ Date _____

Instructor _____ Date _____

PERFORMANCE CHECKLIST 41-3 POUCHING A COLOSTOMY OR ILEOSTOMY

Steps	S	U	Comments
1. Assess existing bag.			
2. Note amount of drainage from stoma.			
3. Assess skin around stoma.			
4. Collect appropriate equipment.			
5. Explain procedure.			
6. Position client.			
7. Wash hands and apply gloves.			
8. Provide privacy.			
9. Remove old appliance as one piece.			
10. Wash skin; dry.			
11. Prepare paste-type barrier if abdominal contour is irregular.			
12. Prepare skin barrier.			
a. Use skin sealant or karaya paste.			
b. Cut hole in barrier.			
c. Cut radial slits from center of hole.			
d. Cut rounded corners on edges of barrier.			
13. Prepare ostomy pouch.			
14. Apply barrier and pouch.			
15. Fold edges of pouch to fit clamp and secure.			
16. Dispose of old appliance.			
17. Remove and dispose of gloves.			
18. Wash hands.			
19. Record pertinent information.			

Student _____ Date _____

Instructor _____ Date _____

PERFORMANCE CHECKLIST 41-4 IRRIGATING A COLOSTOMY

Steps	S	U	Comments
1. Assess stool.	_____	_____	
2. Assess client's understanding of procedure.	_____	_____	
3. Collect appropriate equipment.	_____	_____	
4. Explain procedure.	_____	_____	
5. Assist client with positioning.	_____	_____	
6. Wash hands and apply gloves.	_____	_____	
7. Provide privacy.	_____	_____	
8. Remove appliance and cleanse skin.	_____	_____	
9. Apply irrigation sleeve.	_____	_____	
10. Fill container with solution; hang at client's shoulder level.	_____	_____	
11. Attach cone to irrigating tube.	_____	_____	
12. Apply lubricant to tube.	_____	_____	
13. Insert cone through top of sleeve and then firmly into stoma.	_____	_____	
14. Begin flow and readjust position of cone as needed.	_____	_____	
15. Adjust flow by raising or lowering container.	_____	_____	
16. Administer 500 to 1000 ml of solution slowly over 15 minutes.	_____	_____	
17. When done, clamp tubing and remove cone.	_____	_____	
18. Clamp top of sleeve.	_____	_____	
19. When most of solution has returned, rinse sleeve with water, fold end up, and fasten it to top; have client ambulate, unless restricted to bed.	_____	_____	
20. When all feces returns, rinse sleeve with water and special liquid cleanser.	_____	_____	
21. Remove sleeve and wash sleeve, rinse, and dry.	_____	_____	
22. Apply new pouch.	_____	_____	
23. Dispose of equipment and gloves.	_____	_____	
24. Wash hands.	_____	_____	
25. Inspect volume and character of fecal material.	_____	_____	
26. Note client's response during infusion.	_____	_____	
27. Palpate and auscultate abdomen after return of irrigant.	_____	_____	
28. Record pertinent information.	_____	_____	

Student _____ Date _____

Instructor _____ Date _____

PERFORMANCE CHECKLIST 42-1 **APPLYING RESTRAINTS**

Steps	S	U	Comments
1. Identify client in need of restraint.	————	————	
2. Check physician's order and assess type of restraint needed.	————	————	
3. Explain reason and procedure to client and family.	————	————	
4. Prepare needed equipment.	————	————	
5. Wash hands.	————	————	
6. Apply selected restraint properly, padding bony prominences before applying restraint.	————	————	
7. Secure restraints so they cannot be undone by client.	————	————	
8. Remove restraints properly at appropriate intervals.	————	————	
9. For clients in bed, restraints should be attached to bed frame.	————	————	
10. Wash hands.	————	————	
11. Assess for potential injury to musculoskeletal system at appropriate intervals; observe color of extremity and palpate pulses below extremity.	————	————	
12. Observe for correct application of restraint at appropriate intervals.	————	————	
13. Record procedure and nursing assessment.	————	————	

Student _____ Date _____

Instructor _____ Date _____

PERFORMANCE CHECKLIST 42-2 INTERVENING IN ACCIDENTAL POISONINGS

Steps	S	U	Comments
1. Identify type and amount of substance ingested.	_____	_____	
2. Call poison control center.	_____	_____	
3. Induce vomiting properly if instructed to do so; repeat once if vomiting does not occur in 15 to 20 minutes.	_____	_____	
4. If instructed, save vomitus to deliver to poison control center.	_____	_____	
5. Place victim with head turned to side.	_____	_____	
6. If instructed, call ambulance.	_____	_____	

Student _____ Date _____

Instructor _____ Date _____

PERFORMANCE CHECKLIST 43-1 **PERFORMING PROPER LIFTING**

Steps	S	U	Comments
1. Assess position of weight, height of object, body position, and maximum weight.	_____	_____	
2. Lift object correctly from below center of gravity.			
a. Position your body close to object.	_____	_____	
b. Enlarge your base of support.	_____	_____	
c. Lower your center of gravity to object.	_____	_____	
d. Maintain alignment of head and neck with vertebrae.	_____	_____	
3. Lift object from shelf above center of gravity.			
a. Use safe step stool.	_____	_____	
b. Stand close to shelf.	_____	_____	
c. Quickly transfer weight of object from shelf to arms and over base of support.	_____	_____	

Student _____ Date _____

Instructor _____ Date _____

PERFORMANCE CHECKLIST 43-2 POSITIONING CLIENTS IN BED

Steps	S	U	Comments
1. Assess client's body alignment and comfort level while lying down.	_____	_____	
2. Prepare needed equipment and supplies.	_____	_____	
3. Raise bed to comfortable working height.	_____	_____	
4. Remove all pillows and devices used in previous position.	_____	_____	
5. Recruit extra help as needed.	_____	_____	
6. Explain procedure to client.	_____	_____	
7. Wash hands.	_____	_____	
8. Provide privacy.	_____	_____	
9. Put bed in flat position.	_____	_____	
10. Move client up to head of bed.	_____	_____	
11. Positioning client in supported Fowler's position:			
a. Elevate head of bed 45 to 65 degrees.	_____	_____	
b. Rest head against mattress or small pillow.	_____	_____	
c. If necessary, use pillows to support arms and hands.	_____	_____	
d. Position pillow at lower back.	_____	_____	
e. Place small pillow or roll under thighs and ankles.	_____	_____	
f. Place footboard at bottom of feet.	_____	_____	
12. Positioning hemiplegic client in supported Fowler's position:			
a. Elevate head of bed 45 to 60 degrees.	_____	_____	
b. Sit client up as straight as possible.	_____	_____	
c. Position head with chin slightly forward.	_____	_____	
d. Provide support for involved arm and hand on overbed table in front of client; place arm away from client's side and support elbow with pillow.	_____	_____	
e. Position flaccid hand in normal resting position with wrist slightly extended, arches of hand maintained, fingers partially flexed.	_____	_____	
f. Position spastic hand with wrist in neutral or slightly extended position; fingers should be extended with palm down or in relaxed position with palm up.	_____	_____	
g. Flex knees and hips with pillow or folded blanket under knees.	_____	_____	
h. Support feet in dorsiflexion with footboard or soft pillow.	_____	_____	
13. Positioning client in supine position:			
a. Place client on back with head of bed flat.	_____	_____	
b. Place small rolled towel under lumbar spine.	_____	_____	
c. Place pillow under shoulders, neck, and head.	_____	_____	
d. Place trochanter rolls or sandbags parallel to lateral surface of thighs.	_____	_____	
e. Place small pillow or roll under ankles.	_____	_____	
f. Place footboard against bottom of feet.	_____	_____	
g. Place pillows under pronated forearms, upper arms parallel to body.	_____	_____	
h. Place handrolls in hands.	_____	_____	
14. Positioning hemiplegic client in supine position:			
a. Place head of bed flat.	_____	_____	
b. Place folded towel or pillow under shoulder on affected side.	_____	_____	

   c. Keep affected arm away from body, elbow extended and palm up; or arm out to side with elbow bent, hand toward head of bed. _____ _____

   d. Place affected hand in recommended position for flaccid or spastic hand. _____ _____

   e. Place folded towel under affected hip. _____ _____

   f. Flex affected knee 30 degrees by supporting it on pillow or folded blanket. _____ _____

   g. Support feet with soft pillows at right angle to leg. _____ _____

15. Positioning client in prone position:

   a. Roll client over with arm positioned close to body, elbow straight, and hand under hip. _____ _____

   b. Position client on abdomen in center of bed. _____ _____

   c. Turn head to one side and support with small pillow. _____ _____

   d. Place small pillow under abdomen below level of diaphragm. _____ _____

   e. Support arms in flexed position level at shoulders. _____ _____

   f. Support lower legs with pillow to elevate toes or let toes hang over edge of mattress. _____ _____

16. Positioning hemiplegic client in prone position:

   a. Move client toward unaffected side. _____ _____

   b. Roll client onto side. _____ _____

   c. Place pillow on abdomen. _____ _____

   d. Roll client onto abdomen by positioning involved arm close to body with elbow straight and hand under hip. Roll client over arm. _____ _____

   e. Turn head toward affected side. _____ _____

   f. Position involved arm out to side with elbow bent and hand toward head of bed, fingers extended if possible. _____ _____

   g. Flex both knees slightly by placing pillow under legs. _____ _____

   h. Keep feet at right angles to legs with pillow high enough to keep toes off mattress. _____ _____

17. Positioning client in side-lying (lateral) position:

   a. Lower head of bed as far as tolerated. _____ _____

   b. Position client to one side of bed. _____ _____

   c. Turn client onto side. _____ _____

   d. Place pillow under head and neck. _____ _____

   e. Bring shoulder blade forward. _____ _____

   f. Position arms in slightly flexed position. Upper arm is supported by pillow level with shoulder, other arm by mattress. _____ _____

   g. Place tuck-back pillow behind back. _____ _____

   h. Place pillow under semiflexed upper leg level at hip from groin to foot. _____ _____

   i. Place sandbag parallel to plantar surface of dependent foot. _____ _____

18. Positioning client in Sims' position:

   a. Place head of bed flat. _____ _____

   b. Place client in supine position. _____ _____

   c. Position client in lateral position lying partially on abdomen. _____ _____

   d. Place small pillow under head. _____ _____

   e. Place pillow under flexed upper arm, supporting leg level with hip. _____ _____

   g. Place sandbags parallel to plantar surface of foot. _____ _____

19. Wash hands. _____ _____

20. Observe client's body alignment, level of comfort, and potential pressure points. _____ _____

21. Record procedure in nurses' notes. _____ _____

Student _____ Date _____

Instructor _____ Date _____

PERFORMANCE CHECKLIST 43-3 **MOVING CLIENTS UP IN BED**

Steps	S	U	Comments
1. Assess client's comfort level, activity tolerance, muscle strength, and mobility.	_____	_____	
2. Raise bed to comfortable working height.	_____	_____	
3. Remove pillows and devices previously used.	_____	_____	
4. Recruit extra help as needed.	_____	_____	
5. Explain procedure to client.	_____	_____	
6. Wash hands.	_____	_____	
7. Provide privacy.	_____	_____	
8. Put bed in flat position with wheels on bed locked.	_____	_____	
9. Moving helpless client up in bed (one nurse):			
a. Place client on back with head of bed flat; stand at side of bed.	_____	_____	
b. Place pillow at head of bed.	_____	_____	
c. Place foot of bed at 45-degree angle. Using forward-backward stance, flex knees and hips to bring your arms level with client's legs; shift your weight from front to back leg and slide client's legs toward head of bed.	_____	_____	
d. Move parallel to client's hips; flex knees and hips as needed to bring your arms level with client's hips.	_____	_____	
e. Slide client's hips toward head of bed.	_____	_____	
f. Move parallel to client's head and shoulders; flex knees and hips as needed to bring arms level with client's body.	_____	_____	
g. Slide your arm closest to head of bed under client's neck, with hand reaching under and supporting shoulder.	_____	_____	
h. Place other arm under chest.	_____	_____	
i. Slide trunk diagonally toward head of bed.	_____	_____	
j. Elevate side rail; lower other side rail.	_____	_____	
k. Repeat procedure, switching sides until client reaches desired height in bed.	_____	_____	
l. Center client in bed, moving body in same three sections.	_____	_____	
10. Assisting a client to move up in bed (one or two nurses):			
a. Place client on back with head of bed flat.	_____	_____	
b. Place pillow at head of bed.	_____	_____	
c. Face head of bed. For two nurses, each should have one arm under shoulders and one under thighs; or have one nurse at upper body and one at lower torso.	_____	_____	
d. Place feet apart in forward-backward stance.	_____	_____	

   e. Have client flex knees with feet flat on bed.

   f. Tell client to flex neck, tilting chin toward chest.

   g. Instruct client to help by pushing with feet on bed.

   h. Flex your knees and hips, bringing forearms closer to level of bed.

   i. Ask client to push with heels and elevate trunk while breathing out, moving toward head of bed on count of three.

   j. On count of three, rock and shift your weight from front to back leg while client pushes with heels and elevates trunk.

11. Realign client in appropriate position.

12. Wash hands.

13. Observe client's body alignment, position, level of comfort, and potential pressure points.

14. Record procedure in nurses' notes.

Student _____ Date _____

Instructor _____ Date _____

PERFORMANCE CHECKLIST 43-4 **PERFORMING TRANSFER TECHNIQUES**

Steps	S	U	Comments
1. Assess client's physiological and cognitive status.	____	____	
2. Prepare needed equipment and supplies.	____	____	
3. Explain procedure.	____	____	
4. Wash hands.	____	____	
5. Assisting client to sitting position in bed:			
a. Place client in supine position.	____	____	
b. Remove all pillows.	____	____	
c. Stand facing head of bed.	____	____	
d. Place feet apart with foot nearer bed behind other foot.	____	____	
e. Place hand farthest from client under shoulders, supporting head and neck.	____	____	
f. Place other hand on bed.	____	____	
g. Raise client to sitting position by shifting your weight from front to back leg.	____	____	
h. Push against bed using arm placed on bed surface.	____	____	
6. Assisting client to sitting position on side of bed:			
a. Place client in side-lying position, facing you on side of bed.	____	____	
b. Raise head of bed as high as client can tolerate.	____	____	
c. Stand opposite client's hips.	____	____	
d. Turn diagonally so you face client and far corner of foot of bed.	____	____	
e. Place feet apart in forward-backward stance.	____	____	
f. Place arm nearer head of bed under shoulders, supporting head and neck.	____	____	
g. Place other arm over thighs.	____	____	
h. Move lower legs and feet over side of bed.	____	____	
i. Pivot toward your rear leg, allowing client's upper legs to swing downward.	____	____	
j. At same time, shift your weight to your rear leg and elevate client.	____	____	
k. Remain in front until client regains balance.	____	____	
l. Lower bed until client's feet touch floor.	____	____	
7. Transferring client from bed to chair:			
a. Help client to sitting position on side of bed. Have chair in position at 45-degree angle to bed.	____	____	
b. Apply transfer belt if necessary.	____	____	
c. Ensure that client has nonskid shoes.	____	____	
d. Spread feet apart.	____	____	
e. Flex hips and knees, aligning your knees with client's.	____	____	
f. Grasp transfer belt from underneath or reach through client's axilla and place hands on client's scapulae.	____	____	
g. Rock client up to standing position on count of three while straightening your hips and legs, keeping knees slightly flexed.	____	____	
h. Maintain stability of weak or paralyzed leg with knee.	____	____	
i. Pivot on foot farther from chair.	____	____	
j. Tell client to use armrests on chair for support.	____	____	
k. Flex your hips and knees while lowering client into chair.	____	____	
l. Assess client for proper alignment for sitting position.	____	____	

8. Performing three-person carry:
   a. Three nurses of equal height stand side by side facing side of client's bed. _____ _____
   b. Each person takes responsibility for one of three areas: head and shoulders, hips, or thighs and ankles. _____ _____
   c. Each nurse assumes wide base of support with foot closer to stretcher in front, knees slightly flexed. _____ _____
   d. Lifters' arms are placed under client's head and shoulders, hips, and thighs and ankles with fingers securely around other side of body. _____ _____
   e. Lifters roll client toward their chests. _____ _____
   f. On count of three, client is lifted and held against nurses' chests. _____ _____
   g. On second count of three, nurses step back and pivot toward stretcher, moving forward if necessary. _____ _____
   h. Gently lower client onto center of stretcher, flexing knees and hips until nurses' elbows are level with edge of stretcher. _____ _____
   i. Assess body alignment, place safety straps across client, and raise side rails. _____ _____
9. Place client in selected position. _____ _____
10. Wash hands. _____ _____
11. Observe client to determine response to transfer, correct body alignment, and pressure points. _____ _____
12. Record procedure in nurses' notes. _____ _____

Student _____ Date _____

Instructor _____ Date _____

PERFORMANCE CHECKLIST 43-5 **APPLYING ELASTIC STOCKINGS**

Steps	S	U	Comments
1. Identify need for elastic stockings.	_____	_____	
2. Prepare needed equipment.	_____	_____	
3. Explain procedure.	_____	_____	
4. Wash hands.	_____	_____	
5. Elevate bed to comfortable position.	_____	_____	
6. Place client in supine position.	_____	_____	
7. Cleanse legs; apply small amount of talcum powder to legs and feet.	_____	_____	
8. Turn elastic stocking inside out.	_____	_____	
9. Place client's toe into foot of elastic stocking, making sure stocking is smooth.	_____	_____	
10. Slide remaining portion of stocking over foot.	_____	_____	
11. Slide stocking up over calf until stocking is completely and smoothly extended.	_____	_____	
12. Instruct client not to roll stockings partially down.	_____	_____	
13. Position client comfortably.	_____	_____	
14. Wash hands.	_____	_____	
15. After 1 hour:			
a. Observe stockings for wrinkles or binding.	_____	_____	
b. Assess capillary refill in toes; palpate pulses in feet.	_____	_____	
16. Remove stockings at least once each shift.	_____	_____	
17. Record procedure in nurses' notes.	_____	_____	

Student _____ Date _____

Instructor _____ Date _____

PERFORMANCE CHECKLIST 44-1 ASSESSING FOR RISK OF PRESSURE ULCER DEVELOPMENT

Steps	S	U	Comments
1. Identify clients at risk for pressure ulcer development.	_____	_____	
2. Assess condition of skin over regions of pressure.	_____	_____	
3. Assess client for additional areas of potential pressure.	_____	_____	
4. Observe client for preferred positions when in bed or chair.	_____	_____	
5. Observe client's mobility and ability to initiate and assist with position changes.	_____	_____	
6. Monitor length of time any area of redness persists.			
a. Determine appropriate turning interval.	_____	_____	
b. Use pressure relief device if indicated.	_____	_____	
7. Obtain nutritional assessment data.	_____	_____	
8. Assess client's and family's understanding of risks for pressure ulcers.	_____	_____	
9. Document assessment findings.	_____	_____	

Student _____ Date _____

Instructor _____ Date _____

PERFORMANCE CHECKLIST 44-2 **PLACING CLIENT ON A SUPPORT SURFACE MATTRESS**

Steps	S	U	Comments
1. Assess condition of client's skin.	_____	_____	
2. Prepare necessary equipment and supplies.	_____	_____	
3. Explain procedure to client.	_____	_____	
4. Wash hands.	_____	_____	
5. Provide client privacy.	_____	_____	
6. Apply support surface to bed.	_____	_____	
7. Flotation pad:			
a. Unroll foam pad fully over bed.	_____	_____	
b. Apply sheet over pad.	_____	_____	
c. Place flotation pad in cut-out portion of foam pad.	_____	_____	
8. Foam mattress:			
a. Unroll foam mattress over bed mattress; with egg-crate variety, peaks should point up.	_____	_____	
b. Apply sheet over mattress.	_____	_____	
9. Air mattress:			
a. Apply deflated mattress flat over bed mattress.	_____	_____	
b. Bring plastic flaps or strips around corners of mattress.	_____	_____	
c. Attach connector on air mattress to inflation device.	_____	_____	
d. Inflate mattress to proper air pressure.	_____	_____	
e. Place sheet smoothly over air mattress.	_____	_____	
f. Check air pumps to be sure pressure cycle alternates.	_____	_____	
10. Sheepskin: apply sheepskin flat over desired area of bed mattress.	_____	_____	
11. Position client as desired over support surface; reposition routinely.	_____	_____	
12. Wash hands.	_____	_____	
13. Inspect skin and bony prominences routinely.	_____	_____	
14. Record procedure in nurses' notes.	_____	_____	

Student _____ Date _____

Instructor _____ Date _____

PERFORMANCE CHECKLIST 44-3 **PLACING CLIENT ON A CLINITRON BED**

Steps	S	U	Comments
1. Assess condition of client's skin.	————	————	
2. Prepare necessary equipment and supplies.	————	————	
3. Explain procedure to client and family.	————	————	
4. Obtain additional personnel if needed.	————	————	
5. Wash hands.	————	————	
6. Provide privacy for client.	————	————	
7. Premedicate client for pain approximately 30 minutes before transfer if necessary.	————	————	
8. Transfer client to bed.	————	————	
9. Turn fluidization cycle on and regulate temperature.	————	————	
10. Position client and perform appropriate range of motion exercises.	————	————	
11. Wash hands.	————	————	
12. Inspect skin periodically.	————	————	
13. Ask if client is experiencing nausea.	————	————	
14. Measure level of consciousness.	————	————	
15. Record procedure in nurses' notes.	————	————	

Student _____ Date _____

Instructor _____ Date _____

PERFORMANCE CHECKLIST 44-4 **TREATING PRESSURE ULCERS**

Steps	S	U	Comments
1. Wash hands; apply gloves.	———	———	
2. Provide privacy for client.	———	———	
3. Position comfortably with pressure ulcer and surrounding skin accessible.	———	———	
4. Assemble supplies at bedside; open sterile packages and topical solution containers.	———	———	
5. Expose ulcer area; keep remaining body parts draped.	———	———	
6. Assess pressure ulcer and surrounding skin.			
a. Note color and appearance.	———	———	
b. Measure diameter of ulcer.	———	———	
c. Measure depth of ulcer using sterile item.	———	———	
d. Measure depth of undermining skin by lateral tissue necrosis.	———	———	
7. Cleanse skin around ulcer.	———	———	
8. Rinse area.	———	———	
9. Gently dry skin.	———	———	
10. Apply sterile gloves.	———	———	
11. Properly cleanse ulcer with normal saline or cleansing agent.	———	———	
12. Apply topical agents if prescribed.			
a. Enzymes:			
(1) Keeping gloves sterile, obtain small amount of enzyme ointment in hand.	———	———	
(2) Soften medication by briskly rubbing in palm of hand.	———	———	
(3) Apply thin, even layer of ointment over necrotic areas.	———	———	
(4) Moisten gauze dressing in saline and apply to ulcer.	———	———	
(5) Cover moistened gauze with dry gauze and secure with tape.	———	———	
b. Antiseptics:			
Superficial ulcers			
(1) Moisten sterile gauze with antiseptic solution and apply to ulcer surface.	———	———	
(2) Leave ulcer open to air.	———	———	
Deep ulcers			
(1) Apply antiseptic ointment to dominant gloved hand and spread ointment in and around ulcer.	———	———	
(2) Apply sterile gauze pad over ulcer and secure with tape.	———	———	
c. Oxidizing agents:			
(1) Spread zinc oxide paste over skin surface around ulcer.	———	———	
(2) Moisten gauze dressing in oxidizing solution and apply on ulcer.	———	———	
(3) Apply dry gauze dressing over ulcer.	———	———	

d. Dextranomer beads:
   (1) Hold container of beads approximately 2.5 cm (1 inch) above site and sprinkle 5 mm diameter layer over wound. _____ _____
   (2) Apply gauze dressing over ulcer. _____ _____
e. Hydrocolloid beads or paste:
   (1) Fill ulcer one half of total depth with hydrocolloid beads or paste. _____ _____
   (2) Cover with hydrocolloid dressing; extend dressing 1 to 1½ inches beyond wound edges. _____ _____
f. Hydrogel agents:

   (1) Cover surface of ulcer with hydrogel using sterile applicator or gloved hand. _____ _____
   (2) Completely cover ulcer with dry, fluffy gauze. _____ _____
13. Reposition client comfortably. _____ _____
14. Remove gloves and dispose of soiled supplies; wash hands. _____ _____
15. Report worsening in ulcer's appearance to nurse in charge or physician. _____ _____
16. Record procedure and appearance of ulcer in nurses' notes. _____ _____

Student _____ Date _____

Instructor _____ Date _____

PERFORMANCE CHECKLIST 47-1 DEMONSTRATING POSTOPERATIVE EXERCISES

Steps	S	U	Comments
1. Assess client for risk of postoperative respiratory complications, ability to cough and breathe deeply, and risk for thrombus formation.	_____	_____	
2. Prepare needed equipment and supplies.	_____	_____	
3. Explain purpose and importance of the exercises.	_____	_____	
4. Diaphragmatic breathing:			
a. Have client sit or stand upright with hands palm down along lower borders of anterior rib cage, tips of third fingers lightly together.	_____	_____	
b. Have client take slow, deep breaths, inhaling through nose.	_____	_____	
c. Tell client downward movement of diaphragm will be felt during inspiration and to avoid using chest and shoulder muscles while breathing.	_____	_____	
d. Have client hold breath to count of three and slowly exhale through mouth.	_____	_____	
e. Repeat exercise three to five times.	_____	_____	
f. Have client practice and explain how often to perform exercise.	_____	_____	
5 Incentive spirometry:			
a. Wash hands.	_____	_____	
b. Position client.	_____	_____	
c. Demonstrate correct use of mouthpiece.	_____	_____	
d. Instruct client on correct technique for inspiration and expiration while using device.	_____	_____	
e. Instruct client to breathe normally for short period.	_____	_____	
f. Have client repeat maneuver until goals are achieved.	_____	_____	
g. Wash hands.	_____	_____	
6. Controlled coughing:			
a. Have client assume an upright position; explain its importance.	_____	_____	
b. Demonstrate coughing; take two slow diaphragmatic breaths, inhaling through nose, exhaling through mouth.	_____	_____	
c. Have client inhale a third breath deeply, hold breath to count of three and cough fully two or three times without inhaling.	_____	_____	
d. Caution client against merely clearing throat.	_____	_____	
e. If surgical incision is in chest or abdominal area, show client how to splint cough with both hands over incision (or with pillow).	_____	_____	
f. Have client practice and explain how often to cough and splint.	_____	_____	
7. Turning:			
a. Have client assume supine position on right side of bed.	_____	_____	
b. Be sure side rails are up.	_____	_____	

   c. Have client place left hand over incisional area for splinting.   _____   _____

   d. Have client keep left leg straight and flex right knee up and over left leg.   _____   _____

   e. Have client grasp side rail on left side of bed with right hand, pull toward left, and roll onto left side.   _____   _____

   f. Teach client when to perform maneuver.   _____   _____

8. Leg exercises:

   a. Place client in supine position.   _____   _____

   b. Explain and demonstrate exercises by using passive range of motion exercises.   _____   _____

   c. Rotate each ankle in complete circle; have client draw imaginary circles with big toe and repeat five times.   _____   _____

   d. Alternate dorsiflexion and plantar flexion of feet.   _____   _____

   e. Continue exercises by alternately flexing and extending knees; repeat five times.   _____   _____

   f. Keeping knees straight, alternately raise each leg straight up from bed surface.   _____   _____

   g. Instruct client when and how often to perform exercises and to coordinate turning and leg exercises with breathing and coughing exercises.   _____   _____

9. Observe ability to perform all exercises.   _____   _____

10. Record procedures and observations.   _____   _____

Student _____ Date _____

Instructor _____ Date _____

PERFORMANCE CHECKLIST 47-2 **PREPARING SKIN FOR SURGERY**

Steps	S	U	Comments
1. Assess client's skin.	_____	_____	
2. Review physician's order for site to shave.	_____	_____	
3. Prepare needed equipment and supplies.	_____	_____	
4. Explain procedure and purpose to client.	_____	_____	
5. Wash hands.	_____	_____	
6. Provide privacy.	_____	_____	
7. Raise bed to high position.	_____	_____	
8. Position client comfortably.	_____	_____	
9. Hair clipping:			
a. Lightly dry area to be shaved with towel.	_____	_____	
b. Hold clippers in dominant hand 1 cm above skin and shave in direction of hair growth, one small area at a time.	_____	_____	
c. Rearrange draping as necessary.	_____	_____	
d. Lightly brush away cut hair with towel.	_____	_____	
e. Clean and dry body crevices.	_____	_____	
10. Wet shave:			
a. Place towel or waterproof pad under body part to be shaved.	_____	_____	
b. Drape client, leaving only shaving site exposed.	_____	_____	
c. Adjust lamp.	_____	_____	
d. Lather skin with gauze sponges dipped in antiseptic soap.	_____	_____	
e. Shave one small area of skin at a time; stabilize skin with nondominant hand.	_____	_____	
f. Hold razor at 45-degree angle with dominant hand; shave in direction of hair growth with short, gentle strokes.	_____	_____	
g. Rinse razor as hair accumulates.	_____	_____	
h. Discard blades as they become dull.	_____	_____	
i. Rearrange draping as needed.	_____	_____	
j. Use washcloth and warm water to rinse remaining soap from skin. Change water as needed.	_____	_____	
k. Cleanse and dry body crevices.	_____	_____	
l. Discard waterproof pad or towel.	_____	_____	
m. Observe for nicks in skin.	_____	_____	
11. Tell client procedure is over.	_____	_____	
12. Clean and dispose of equipment and supplies.	_____	_____	
13. Wash hands.	_____	_____	
14. Inspect condition of skin.	_____	_____	
15. Record procedure and observations.	_____	_____	

PERFORMANCE CHECKLIST 47-3 **MAINTAINING AN NG TUBE**

Steps	S	U	Comments
1. Assess client's oral cavity.	____	____	
2. Palpate abdomen.	____	____	
3. Check medical record.	____	____	
4. Prepare needed equipment and supplies at bedside.	____	____	
5. Identify client and explain procedure.	____	____	
6. Wash hands and apply gloves.	____	____	
7. Position client and raise bed to highest horizontal level.	____	____	
8. Place equipment on side of bed nearest nurse.	____	____	
9. Provide privacy.	____	____	
10. Stand on right side of bed if right-handed; left side if left-handed.	____	____	
11. Place bath towel over chest.	____	____	
12. Keep facial tissues within reach.	____	____	
13. Instruct client to breathe normally, and occlude one naris at a time to select nostril with greater airflow.	____	____	
14. Measure distance to insert tube by extending tube from nose to tip of earlobe and down to xiphoid process or by using Hanson method.	____	____	
15. Mark length of tube to be inserted.	____	____	
16. Cut 10 cm of tape and split one end lengthwise 5 cm.	____	____	
17. Curve 10 to 15 cm of tube tightly around index finger, then release.	____	____	
18. Lubricate 7.5 to 10 cm of end of tube with water-soluble lubricating jelly.	____	____	
19. Ask client to extend neck and insert tube slowly through naris with curved end pointing downward.	____	____	
20. Continue to pass tube along floor of nasal passage, applying gentle pressure if mild resistance is felt, but do not force.	____	____	
21. Withdraw tube if resistance is felt; begin again with other naris.	____	____	
22. Continue insertion until just past nasopharynx. Stop tube advancement to allow client to relax; provide tissues. Tell client that next step requires swallowing.	____	____	
23. With tube just above oropharynx, ask client to flex head forward and dry swallow or suck in air through straw; advance tube 2.5 to 5 cm with each swallow.	____	____	
24. If client has trouble swallowing and can take fluids, offer glass of water.	____	____	
25. If client begins to cough, gag, or choke, stop advancing tube until client breathes easily; offer another sip of water.	____	____	
26. Withdraw tube slightly if client continues coughing.	____	____	
27. If gagging continues, check back of pharynx.	____	____	
28. After client relaxes, continue to advance tube desired distance.	____	____	
29. Checking tube placement:			
a. Ask client to talk.	____	____	
b. Check tube placement.	____	____	
c. Attach syringe to tube and aspirate gently back on syringe to obtain gastric contents.	____	____	
d. If tube is not in stomach, advance another 2.5 to 5 cm and again check tube position.	____	____	

30. Anchoring tube:
    a. Clamp end of tube or connect to drainage bag or suction machine. _____ _____
    b. Properly tape tube to nose, avoiding pressure on naris. _____ _____
    c. Fasten end of tube to gown. _____ _____
    d. Elevate head of bed unless ordered otherwise. _____ _____
    e. Reassure client that sensation will diminish. _____ _____
    f. Record procedure. _____ _____
31. Performing tube irrigation:
    a. Check tube placement. _____ _____
    b. Draw 30 ml of normal saline in appropriate syringe. _____ _____
    c. Clamp tubing proximal to connection site of drainage or suction apparatus. _____ _____
    d. Disconnect tubing and lay end on towel. _____ _____
    e. Insert tip of syringe into end of tube. _____ _____
    f. Inject saline slowly and evenly; do not force solution. _____ _____
    g. If resistance occurs, check for kinks in tubing; report repeated resistance to physician. _____ _____
    h. After instilling saline, immediately aspirate to withdraw fluid. _____ _____
    i. Measure volume of liquid aspirated. _____ _____
    j. Reconnect tube to drainage or suction; if solution does not return, repeat irrigation. _____ _____
    k. Record each irrigation. _____ _____
32. Discontinuing NG tube:
    a. Apply nonsterile gloves. _____ _____
    b. Turn off suction and disconnect tube from drainage tube or bag. _____ _____
    c. Remove tape from nose and unpin tube from gown. _____ _____
    d. Explain procedure and reassure client. _____ _____
    e. Give client facial tissue and place towel across chest. _____ _____
    f. Tell client to take deep breath and hold. _____ _____
    g. Clamp or kink tubing and pull tube steadily as client holds breath. _____ _____
    h. Dispose of tube and drainage equipment. _____ _____
    i. Measure drainage. _____ _____
    j. Change gloves if necessary. _____ _____
    k. Clean nares and provide mouth care. _____ _____
    l. Position client comfortably and explain procedure for drinking fluids. _____ _____
    m. Clean equipment; properly dispose of soiled linen. _____ _____
    n. Remove and dispose of gloves. Wash hands. _____ _____
    o. Observe contents of NG tube. _____ _____
    p. Palpate abdomen. _____ _____
    q. Inspect nares and nose. _____ _____
    r. Record procedure and observations. _____ _____

Student _____ Date _____

Instructor _____ Date _____

PERFORMANCE CHECKLIST 48-1 APPLYING DRY AND WET-TO-DRY DRESSINGS

Steps	S	U	Comments
1. Assess wound and client's comfort level.	_____	_____	
2. Review medical orders.	_____	_____	
3. Prepare needed equipment and supplies.	_____	_____	
4. Explain procedure and purpose to client.	_____	_____	
5. Instruct client not to touch wound area or sterile supplies.	_____	_____	
6. Provide privacy and close windows.	_____	_____	
7. Position client comfortably.	_____	_____	
8. Drape client with bath blanket, exposing only wound site.	_____	_____	
9. Wash hands.	_____	_____	
10. Make cuff at top of disposable bag and place nearby.	_____	_____	
11. Apply gloves.	_____	_____	
12. Remove tape of previous dressing by gently pulling parallel to skin and toward dressing.	_____	_____	
13. Remove adhesive left on skin.	_____	_____	
14. With gloved hand or forceps, remove dressing, keeping soiled surface away from client. If wet-to-dry dressing sticks, gently free dressing; warn client of discomfort and do not moisten dressing.	_____	_____	
15. Observe character and amount of drainage on dressing.	_____	_____	
16. Properly dispose of dressings.	_____	_____	
17. Properly remove and dispose of gloves.	_____	_____	
18. Open sterile dressing tray or individually wrapped sterile supplies. Place on bedside table.	_____	_____	
19. Dry dressing:			
a. Pour antiseptic solution into sterile basin or over sterile gauze.	_____	_____	
b. Apply sterile gloves.	_____	_____	
c. Insert wound for appearance, drains, and integrity.	_____	_____	
d. Cleanse wound with antiseptic solution, using separate swab for each stroke, cleaning from least contaminated to most contaminated area.	_____	_____	
e. Swab the wound area with dry gauze.	_____	_____	
f. Apply antiseptic ointment if ordered.	_____	_____	
g. Apply dry sterile dressings to incision or wound site; begin with contact layer. Cut 4 × 4 gauze to fit around drain; apply second layer of gauze, and apply surgical pad.	_____	_____	
20. Wet-to-dry dressing:			
a. Pour solution into sterile basin; add fine-mesh gauze.	_____	_____	
b. Apply sterile gloves.	_____	_____	
c. Inspect wound condition.	_____	_____	
d. Cleanse wound with prescribed antiseptic or normal saline from least to most contaminated area.	_____	_____	

   e. Apply moist fine-mesh gauze onto wound, ensuring all
      surfaces are in contact with moist gauze.   ———————   ———————
   f. Apply dry sterile 4 × 4 over wet gauze.   ———————   ———————
   g. Cover with ABD pad, surgi-pad, or gauze.   ———————   ———————
21. Properly apply tape, Kling roll, or Montgomery ties over
    dressing.   ———————   ———————
22. Properly remove and dispose of gloves.   ———————   ———————
23. Assist client to comfortable position.   ———————   ———————
24. Dispose of all supplies.   ———————   ———————
25. Wash hands.   ———————   ———————
26. Reassess client.   ———————   ———————
27. Monitor dressing status at least every shift.   ———————   ———————
28. Record procedure and observations.   ———————   ———————

Student _____ Date _____

Instructor _____ Date _____

PERFORMANCE CHECKLIST 48-2 PERFORMING WOUND IRRIGATION

Steps	S	U	Comments
1. Review medical record and recent recordings of wound.	————	————	
2. Assess client's comfort level.	————	————	
3. Properly administer prescribed analgesic before irrigation.	————	————	
4. Prepare needed equipment and supplies at bedside.	————	————	
5. Explain procedure.	————	————	
6. Position client so irrigating solution flows from upper end of wound into collection basin.	————	————	
7. Warm irrigating solution properly.	————	————	
8. Prepare leakproof refuse bag.	————	————	
9. Provide privacy.	————	————	
10. Place waterproof pad on bed in front of wound and place basin under wound.	————	————	
11. Wash hands.	————	————	
12. Apply gown if needed.	————	————	
13. Prepare sterile field using dressing set and supplies.	————	————	
14. Prepare sterile basin with irrigating solution and syringe.	————	————	
15. Place tape strips within reach but off sterile field.	————	————	
16. Apply clean gloves.	————	————	
17. Remove and discard soiled dressing properly.	————	————	
18. Remove soiled gloves.	————	————	
19. Inspect wound.	————	————	
20. Apply sterile gloves.	————	————	
21. To irrigate wound with wide opening:			
a. Fill syringe with irrigating solution.	————	————	
b. Hold syringe 2.5 cm above upper end of wound.	————	————	
c. Flush wound properly.	————	————	
d. Repeat until solution draining into basin is clear.	————	————	
22. To irrigate deep wound with very small opening:			
a. Attach soft catheter to filled syringe.	————	————	
b. Lubricate tip of catheter and insert gently into wound.	————	————	
c. Flush wound properly.	————	————	
d. Pinch off catheter below syringe.	————	————	
e. Fill syringe; reattach to catheter; repeat until return is clear.	————	————	
23. Dry wound edges with sterile gauze.	————	————	
24. Apply sterile dressing.	————	————	
25. Remove gloves.	————	————	
26. Secure dressing with tape.	————	————	
27. Assist client to comfortable position.	————	————	
28. Dispose of equipment and refuse bag properly.	————	————	
29. Wash hands.	————	————	
30. Inspect dressing periodically.	————	————	
31. Evaluate skin integrity.	————	————	
32. Record procedure and observations.	————	————	

Student _____ Date _____
Instructor _____ Date _____

PERFORMANCE CHECKLIST 48-3 APPLYING AN ABDOMINAL BINDER, T BINDER, OR BREAST BINDER

Steps	S	U	Comments
1. Assess client's ability to breathe deeply and cough effectively.			
2. Assess client's skin integrity.			
3. Review medical record.			
4. Determine appropriate binder.			
5. Prepare needed equipment and supplies at bedside.			
6. Explain procedure and purpose to client.			
7. Wash hands.			
8. Provide privacy.			
9. Apply abdominal binder.			
a. Place client in supine position.			
b. Fanfold far side of binder toward midline.			
c. Help client roll away from nurse toward raised side rail while supporting incision with hands.			
d. Place fanfolded ends of binder under client.			
e. Help client roll over folded ends.			
f. Unfold and stretch ends out smoothly on far side of bed.			
g. Have client roll back into supine position.			
h. Center client over binder.			
i. Properly close straight binder.			
j. Assess ability to breathe deeply and cough effectively.			
k. Assess comfort level.			
l. Adjust binder as necessary.			
10. Apply T and double-T binders.			
a. Help client to dorsal recumbent position.			
b. Have client raise hips.			
c. Place horizontal band around waist with vertical tails extending past buttocks.			
d. Overlap waistband in front and secure.			
e. For T binder, bring remaining strip over perineal dressing, up and under front of band; bring ends over waistband and secure. For double-T binder, bring vertical strips over perineal or suprapubic dressing, with each tail supporting one side of scrotum; draw ends behind and downward in front of band and secure.			
f. Assess comfort level; readjust binder and increase padding as needed.			
g. Instruct client about care of binder before and after elimination.			
11. Apply breast binder.			
a. Help client place arms through binder's armholes.			
b. Help client to supine position.			
c. Pad under breasts if necessary.			
d. Secure binder first at nipple level, then above and below until binder is closed.			
e. Adjust binder as necessary for individualized fit.			
f. Observe level of self-care in reapplying binder.			
12. Wash hands.			
13. Assess wound site.			
14. Note comfort level.			
15. Record procedure and observations.			

Student _____ Date _____

Instructor _____ Date _____

PERFORMANCE CHECKLIST 48-4 **APPLYING AN ELASTIC BANDAGE**

Steps	S	U	Comments
1. Assess client's skin integrity and circulation.	_____	_____	
2. Review medical record.	_____	_____	
3. Prepare needed equipment and supplies at bedside.	_____	_____	
4. Explain procedure to client.	_____	_____	
5. Wash hands.	_____	_____	
6. Provide privacy.	_____	_____	
7. Help client to comfortable, correct position.	_____	_____	
8. With roll of bandage in dominant hand, hold beginning of bandage at distal body part with other hand. Continue transferring bandage properly as it is wrapped.	_____	_____	
9. Apply bandage from distal point to proximal boundary using necessary turns.	_____	_____	
10. Unroll and slightly stretch bandage.	_____	_____	
11. Overlap turns.	_____	_____	
12. Secure first bandage before applying additional rolls.	_____	_____	
13. Evaluate distal circulation after application is completed and at least twice during 8-hour period.	_____	_____	
14. Record procedure and observations.	_____	_____	

Student _____ Date _____

Instructor _____ Date _____

PERFORMANCE CHECKLIST 48-5 APPLYING A HOT, MOIST COMPRESS TO AN OPEN WOUND

Steps	S	U	Comments
1. Assess wound.	_____	_____	
2. Assess client's response to temperature and pain.	_____	_____	
3. Review physician's order.	_____	_____	
4. Prepare needed equipment and supplies at bedside.	_____	_____	
5. Explain procedure and purpose to client.	_____	_____	
6. Assist client to comfortable position with proper body alignment.	_____	_____	
7. Place waterproof pad under area to be treated.	_____	_____	
8. Provide privacy.	_____	_____	
9. Drape client with bath blanket, exposing body part to be covered with compresses.	_____	_____	
10. Wash hands.	_____	_____	
11. Assemble equipment, pour warmed solution into sterile container, open sterile packages, and immerse gauze in container.	_____	_____	
12. Apply gloves.	_____	_____	
13. Remove wound dressing properly.	_____	_____	
14. Properly dispose of gloves and dressings.	_____	_____	
15. Assess condition of wound and surrounding skin.	_____	_____	
16. Apply sterile gloves.	_____	_____	
17. Apply sterile petrolatum jelly with cotton swab to skin around wound.	_____	_____	
18. Wring excess water from one layer of immersed gauze.	_____	_____	
19. Apply gauze to open wound. Watch client's response and ask if discomfort is felt.	_____	_____	
20. After a few seconds, lift edge of gauze to assess for redness.	_____	_____	
21. If client tolerates compress, pack gauze snugly against wound, ensuring all wound surfaces are covered.	_____	_____	
22. Wrap moist compress with dry bath towel; tie or pin in place if necessary.	_____	_____	
23. Change hot compress every 5 minutes or as ordered.	_____	_____	
24. (Optional) Apply aquathermic or waterproof heating pad over towel, keeping it in place for duration of procedure.	_____	_____	
25. Ask client periodically if discomfort or burning sensation is felt.	_____	_____	
26. Remove pad, towel, and compress in 30 minutes.	_____	_____	
27. Assess wound and surrounding skin.	_____	_____	
28. Replace dry sterile dressing.	_____	_____	
29. Assist client to comfortable position.	_____	_____	
30. Dispose of equipment and suppliies properly.	_____	_____	
31. Wash hands.	_____	_____	
32. Inspect affected area.	_____	_____	
33. Ask client about any new burning sensation.	_____	_____	
34. Record procedure and observations.	_____	_____	